Question Bank of Veterinary Gynaecology Obstetrics and Andrology

Question Bank of Veterinary Gynaecology Obstetrics and Andrology

By :

Dr. Matendra Singh Thakur
Professor & I/C Head of Veterinary Gynaecology & Obstetrics
College of Veterinary Science & A.H., Rewa (M.P.)
Nanaji Deshmukh Veterinary Science University, Jabalpur (M.P.)

Dr. Suresh Prasad Shukla
Dean & Professor
College of Veterinary Science & A.H., Rewa (M.P.)
Nanaji Deshmukh Veterinary Science University, Jabalpur (M.P.)

Dr. Madhu Shivhare
Teaching Associate
College of Veterinary Science & A.H., Rewa (M.P.)
Nanaji Deshmukh Veterinary Science University, Jabalpur (M.P.)

SSPH

SATISH SERIAL PUBLISHING HOUSE
403, Express Tower, Commercial Complex, Azadpur, Delhi-110033 (India)
Phone : 011-27672852, Fax : 91-11-27672046
E-mail : info@satishserial.com, hkjain1975@yahoo.com
Website : www.satishserial.com

Published by :

SATISH SERIAL PUBLISHING HOUSE
403, Express Tower, Commercial Complex, Azadpur, Delhi-110033 (INDIA)
Phone : 011-27672852 Fax : 91-11-27672046
E-mail : info@satishserial.com, hkjain1975@yahoo.com

ISBN 978-93-85055-28-7

Typeset at: Harminder Kharb *for* Laxmi Art Creation
Printed at: Salasar Imaging Systems, Delhi-110035

PREFACE

Multiple choice questions offer students good scoring system to boost their performance ,deep knowledge and understanding of the subject is a pre requisite for solving the multiple choice question & therefore reverse, also holds good in that multiple choice question provide knowledge in depth of the subject studied.

An attempt has been made by the author cum editors to provide maximum possible question in this format to help the readers to obtain thorough knowledge of the subject covering all the course of the veterinary gynaecology & obstetrics as per syllabus of Veterinary Council of India (VCI).

This multi author question bank book hopefully will be very useful to undergraduate(UG) and postgraduate (PG) students of veterinary gynaecology & obstetrics not only in scoring marks but also in solving field oriented problems faced by them.

All possible attempts have been made in maintaining clarity and uniqueness of answers still, we welcome suggestion to overcome ambiguity if forward in any of the multiple choice question.

M.S. Thakur
S.P. Shukla
Madhu Shivhare

CONTENTS

Questions and Answers ???

Gynaecology

1) Maternal recognition of pregnancy in cattle occurs between the -
   (a) 10-12 days of gestation (b) 15-17 days of gestation
   (c) 20-23 days of gestation (d) 30-35 days of gestation

2) The corpus luteum of pregnancy is known as –
   (a) Corpus luteum albicans (b) Persistant corpus luteum
   (c) Corpus luteum verum (d) Cystic corpora lutea

3) Oviductal secretions are regulated by -
   (a) Ovarian Steriod Hormone (b) FSH
   (c) LH (d) Inhibin

4) Protein B hormone is secreted from -
   (a) Uterus (b) Hypothalamus
   (c) Placenta (d) Adenohypophysis

5) Androgens are produced by -
   (a) Lutein cells (b) Leydig cells
   (c) Sertoli cells (d) Theca interna cells

6) In aging females early embryonic mortality may be due to -
   (a) Poor egg quality (b) High rise of temperature.
   (c) Sub oestrus (d) Over feeding

7) Bartlett technique is used for the diagnosis of -
   (a) Brucellosis (b) Tubal patency
   (c) Trichomoniasis (d) Leptospirosis

8) FSHP can be used for -
(a) Oestrus synchronization (b) Induction of parturition
(c) Super ovulation (d) Treatment of luteal cyst

9) In cattle the fertile life of ova is -
(a) 10-15 hrs (b) 20-25 hrs
(c) 30-48 hrs (d) 70-80 hrs

10) In swine the fertile life of ova -
(a) 8-10 hrs (b) 20-30 hrs
(c) 30-40 hrs (d) 50-60 hrs

11) Pig blastocyst begins to attach to the uterine surface on day-
(a) 7 (b) 13
(c) 20 (d) 30

12) In the mare implantation does not occur until days -
(a) 5-10 (b) 10-15
(c) 15-20 (d) 25-30

13) In sheep the average gestation period is -
(a) 114 days (b) 148 days
(c) 180 days (d) 210 days

14) The equine chorionic gonadotrophin is secreted from -
(a) Trophoblastic cells (b) Endometrium
(c) Corpus luteum (d) Theca interns cells

15) In case of cows the longest phase of oestrus cycle is -
(a) Proestrus (b) Oestrus
(c) Metoestrus (d) Diestrus

16) The anterior part of vagina which develops into a pouch /pocket around the cervix known as -
(a) Bursa (b) Vestibule
(c) Fornix (d) Diverticulum

17) Mibolerone is a -
(a) Synthetic oestrogen (b) Synthetic androgen
(c) Synthetic progesterone (d) Synthetic PGF_2 alpha

18) Pseudo pregnancy may occur as a result of increased concentration of -

(a) FSH (b) LH
(c) Oxytocin (d) Prolactin

19) Tranmissible venereal tumor is commonly seen in -

(a) Bitches (b) Cows
(c) Sheep (d) Mares

20) Commercially available preparation of GnRH is -

(a) Fertagyl (b) Illirin
(c) Crestar (d) Progynon Depot

21) Lutinizing hormones can be used for the treatment of -

(a) Anovulation (b) Genital prolapse
(c) Anoestrus (d) Pyometra

22) Synchronization of the oestrus cycle in cyclic animals involves administration of -

(a) FSH (b) LH
(c) PGF_2 alpha (d) Estrogen

23) Vaginal mucus impedance can be used for -

(a) Estrus detection (b) Diagnosis of COD
(c) Diagnosis of Brucellosis (d) Diagnosis of Trichomoniasis

24) In bitches the duration of estrus is -

(a) 1-2 days (b) 2-3 days
(c) 3-5 days (d) 4-7 days

25) Stimulation of cervix is essential for ovulation in -

(a) Buffalo (b) Mare
(c) Rabbit (d) Cow

26) Anovulatory estrus is more common in -

(a) Swine (b) Sheep
(c) Cattle (d) Bitch

27) In mares Cuboni test can be performed for pregnancy diagnosis during -

(a) 60-80 days (b) 80-120 days
(c) 150-200 days (d) 200-300 days

28) The shape of ovary is Bean shaped in -

(a) Cow (b) Buffalo
(c) Mare (d) Sheep

29) In India the most common cause of anoestrus is -

(a) Nutritional deficiency (b) Hormonal Imbalance
(c) Over feeding (d) Genetic causes

30) Prostaglandin F2 alpha is a –

(a) Protein hormone (b) Steroid hormone
(c) Local hormone (d) None of the above

31) T shaped uterus is found in –

(a) Mare (b) Cow
(c) Bitch (d) Sow

32) The largest size of the uterine horn is found in –

(a) Buffalo (b) Cow
(c) Mare (d) Sow

33) The largest size of clitoris is observed in –

(a) Mare (b) Cow
(c) Bitch (d) Sow

34) Ovulation in cattle occurs -

(a) During mid estrus
(b) Occurs after mating only
(c) Before the end of oestrus
(d) 12-14 hrs after the end of oestrus

35) During luteal phase the level of the following is increased -

(a) Cortisol (b) Estradiol
(c) Progesterone (d) Adrenalin

36) Photoperiodism is characteristic of the reproductive cycle of -

(a) Cow (b) Cat
(c) Bitch (d) Sheep

37) The hormone PMSG is produced in pregnant mare at -

(a) 10-15 days (b) 20-30 days
(c) 40-120 days (d) 150-200 days

38) Super ovulation in cattle involves stimulation of multiple follicular development using hormone-

(a) Estrogen (b) Progesterone
(c) LH (d) FSH

39) At birth each 0vary may contain primary follicles upto-

(a) 100 (b) 1000
(c) 10000 (d) More than 100000

40) The normal life span of corpus luteum is unaltered in the absence of uterus in case of –

(a) Bitch (b) Sheep
(c) Mare (d) Sow

41) The luteolytic action of the uterine horn is directed exclusively to the corpus luteum on the adjacent ovary in case of –

(a) Mare (b) Cow
(c) Sow (d) Bitch

42) During oestrus repeated exposure of the clitoris is observed in –

(a) Sheep (b) Mare
(c) Cow (d) Sow

43) The fertile life of ovum in the genital tract of mare is –

(a) 6-8 hours (b) 10-15 hours
(c) 20-24 hours (d) 30-40 hours

44) The fertile life of ovum in the genital tract of sheep is –

(a) 5-10 hours (b) 16-24 hours
(c) 30-35 hours (d) 40-50 hours

45) The secretions of gonadotrophin is regulated by –
(a) Pituitary gland (b) Hypothalamus
(c) Ovary (d) All of the above

46) The life span of corpus luteum is similar in pregnant and non pregnant females in –
(a) Mare (b) Sow
(c) Kangaroo (d) Cat

47) The length of gestation is similar to that of the estrous cycle in –
(a) Bitch (b) Cat
(c) Opossum (d) Sheep

48) The neonates are born blind in –
(a) Cattle (b) Sheep
(c) Dog (d) Sow

49) The PMSG is in effective and will not cause super ovulation in –
(a) Cow (b) Buffalo
(c) Mare (d) Ewe

50) Placental lactogen is a-
(a) Para hormone (b) Protein hormone
(c) Steroid hormone (d) None

51) Short acting corticosteroids can be used for -
(a) Induction of estrous (b) Treatment of cystic ovaries
(c) Induction of parturition (d) None

52) Folltrophin can be used for –
(a) Induction of parturition (b) Oestrus synchronization
(c) Super ovulation (d) None

53) Rough rasp like corrugations on the vaginal mucosa is the pathognomic lesion of –
(a) Brucellosis (b) Vibriosis
(c) Trichomoniasis (d) Leptospirosis

54) Bangs disease is also known as -
(a) Vibriosis (b) Brucellosis
(c) Leptspirosis (d) Trichomoniasis

55) Scheim Zondeck test can be used for pregnancy diagnosis in -
(a) Bitch (b) Mare
(c) Cow (d) Sow

56) Cuboni test can be used for pregnancy diagnosis in-
(a) Buffalo (b) Cow
(c) Mare (d) Sow

57) Melengesterol acetate is a synthetic -
(a) Oestrogen (b) Progesterone
(c) PGF2 alpha (d) Gonadotropin

58) HGC hormone is secreted from -
(a) Ovary (b) Human placenta
(c) Pituitary gland (d) Hypothalamus

59) Fremitus can be used as diagnostic tool for the diagnosis of -
(a) Uterine torsion (b) Overo- bursal adhesion
(c) Dead fetus (d) None

60) Progesterone is secreted from -
(a) Uterus (b) Corpus luteum
(c) Follicle (d) Pituitary gland

61) The estrogen is secreted from -
(a) Corpus luteum (b) Endometrium
(c) Theca interna cells (d) Uterus

62) Estradiol 17 beta at estrous -
(a) Facilitate removal of micro-organism
(b) Favours establishment of uterine infection
(c) Facilitates accumulation of pus
(d) None

63) The local production of antibodies in the reproductive tract is regulated by-
(a) Ovarian steroid hormones (b) GnRH
(c) PGF_2 alpha (d) None

64) The PMSG is secreted from
(a) Ovary (b) Hypothalamus
(c) Pituitary gland (d) Equine placenta

65) Barker,s syndrome is associated with necrosis of -
(a) Liver (b) Lung
(c) Cerebral cortex (d) Kideny

66) Split estrous is commonly observed in –
(a) Buffaloes (b) Mare
(c) Bitch (d) Sow

67) The normal gestation length in buffalo is –
(a) 270-280 days (b) 280-290 days
(c) 290- 300 days (d) 300-310 days

68) In case of mares the normal gestation period is –
(a) 290-300 days (b) 300-310days
(c) 330-340 days (d) 360-370 days

69) The normal gestation period in bitch is –
(a) 50-55 days (b) 56-65 days
(c) 65-70 days (d) 70-75 days

70) In camel the normal gestation period is –
(a) 250-275 days (b) 275-300 days
(c) 300-330 day (d) 333-430 days

71) The normal gestation length in sow is –
(a) 70-80 days (b) 90-100 days
(c) 90-100 days (d) 113-115 days

72) In beer the normal gestation length is –
(a) 150-170 days (b) 170-200 days
(c) 200-205 days (d) 208-240 days

73) The normal gestation length in sheep is –
(a) 115-125 days (b) 125-135 days
(c) 140-155 days (d) 160-170 days

74) In lion the normal gestation length is –
(a) 70-80 days (b) 80-90days
(c) 105-112 days (d) 115-120 days

75) In elephant the normal gestation length is -
(a) 400-450 days (b) 500-550 days
(c) 615 -650 days (d) 700-730 days

76) In cattle the maximum early embryonic mortality takes place during the gestation period of -
(a) 4-6 days (b) 8-16 days
(c) 16-25 days (d) 30-35 days

77) The induced ovulation occurs in –
(a) Buffalo (b) Mare
(c) Camel (d) Sow

78) The implantation of the zygote in the endometrium of sheep occurs during gestation period of –
(a) 4-6 days (b) 6-8days
(c) 9-15 days (d) 20-30 days

79) In indigenous female cattle the age at maturity is –
(a) 12 months (b) 18 months
(c) 35 months (d) 60 months

80) In case of bitch the age at maturity is –
(a) 8-10 months (b) 12-18 months
(c) 18-24 months (d) 24-30 months

81) The onset of puberty in mare is –
(a) 6-8 months (b) 10-24 months
(c) 24-30 months (d) 30-36 months

82) Onset of puberty in sow is –
(a) 5-8 months (b) 8-12 months
(c) 12-18 months (d) 18-24 months

83) In mare ovulation occurs during –
(a) 1-2 days during oestrus (b) 1-2 days before end of oestrus
(c) After oestrus (d) None

84) Optimum time for service in sow is –
(a) 5-10 hours after the onset of estrum
(b) 12-30 hours after the onset of estrum
(c) 36-48 hours after the onset of estrum
(d) 50-70 hours after the onset of estrum

85) The length of estrum in bitch is –
(a) 1-4 day (b) 4-13day
(c) 15-18 day (d) 20-24 day

86) The optimum time of service in bitch is –
(a) 1-2 day after the onset of estrum
(b) 4-6 day after the onset of estrum
(c) 1-2 days after the end of estrum
(d) 4-6 days after the end of estrum

87) The average age at first calving in buffaloes is –
(a) 30 months (b) 40 months
(c) 55 months (d) 75 months

88) The average age at maturity in cross-bred cows is –
(a) 12 months (b) 18 months
(c) 30 months (d) 40 months

89) The average age at first calving in Gir cows is –
(a) 25 months (b) 35 months
(c) 45 months (d) 55 months

90) The average age at sexual maturity in Sahiwal cows is –

(a) 18 months (b) 30 months

(c) 40 months (d) 50 months

91) Unfertilized ovum remains for months in the oviduct of – –species

(a) Sow (b) Mare

(c) Ewe and Doe (d) Bitch

92) In sows, maternal recognition of pregnancy is mainly due to the action of

(a) Interferon tau (b) Oxytocin

(c) Estrogen (d) Prostaglandins

93) Ovulation of "primary oocyte" occurs in

(a) Bitch (b) Sow

(c) Cow and doe (d) Mare

94) In case of pregnant mares endometrial cups are formed during-

(a) 1st month of pregnancy

(b) During 2nd month of pregnancy

(c) During 3rd month of pregnancy

(d) During 4th month of pregnancy

95) In case of mares corpus luteum verum can only be palpated per rectum for –

(a) 2-3 days after its formation

(b) 7-8 days after its

(c) 10-12 days after its formation

(d) 15-16 days after its formation

96) For identification of PMSG in the pregnant mares the blood samples should be collected preferably between-

(a) 10-30 days after service (b) 40-120 days after service

(c) 150-200 days after service (d) 200-250 days after service

97) In which species semen is alkaline -

(a) Ram (b) Buck

(c) Boar (d) Bull

98) The time of maternal recognition of pregnancy in ewe is –
(a) 10-11 days (b) 12-13 days
(c) 14-16 days (d) 16- 18 days

99) The time of maternal recognition of pregnancy in sow is –
(a) 10-11 days (b) 12 days
(c) 13-14 days (d) 15-16 days

100) The time of maternal recognition of pregnancy in mare is –
(a) 10-11 days (b) 12-13 days
(c) 14-16 days (d) 18-20 days

101) The day of definite attachment of conceptus in cow is -
(a) 15-20days (b) 25-30 days
(c) 30-35 days (d) 40-45 days

102) The day of definite attachment of conceptus in sow is –
(a) Day 12 (b) Day 15
(c) Day 18 (d) Day 25

103) The day of definite attachment of conceptus in ewe is –
(a) 12-13 days (b) 15-16 days
(c) 25-30days (d) 30-35 days

104) The day of definite attachment of conceptus in mare is –
(a) 10-12 days (b) 15-20days
(c) 25-38 days (d) 40-45 days

105) The epithelial cells that surround the antrum are known as –
(a) Theca cells (b) Lutein cells
(c) Granulosa cells (d) None of the above

106) The half life of the PMSG is more than FSH because of the presence of –
(a) Ascorbic acid (b) Sialic acid
(c) Acetic acid (d) None of the above

107) In cow the stage of blastocyst is -
(a) 3-4 days after ovulation (b) 4-6 days after ovulation
(c) 6-8 days after ovulation (d) 8-10 days after ovulation

108) The interval between two successive heat is known as -
(a) Inter calving period (b) Service period
(c) Post partum period (d) Inter-estrus period

109) The potent analogue of PGF_2 alpha is -
(a) Prigma (b) Estrumate
(c) Dinoprost (d) All of the above

110) Ziel - nelson method of staining can be used for the diagnosis of -
(a) Brucella (b) Trichomonas
(c) Compylobacter (d) None

111) The FSH release is inhibited by -
(a) Adrenalin (b) Inhibin
(c) Dopamine (d) Nor-adrenalin

112) The ACTH is secreted by -
(a) Pituitary gland (b) Adrenal cortex
(c) Adrenal medulla (d) Ovary

113) The secretion of the LH is enhanced by -
(a) Morphin (b) Chlomiphene
(c) Atropin (d) Chlorpromazin

114) The nature of FSH is -
(a) Steroid (b) Glycoprotein
(c) Nucleoprotein (d) None of the above

115) Photoperiodism is a characteristic of the sexual activity in -
(a) Sheep, goat and horse (b) Dog
(c) Cow (d) Sow

116) The effect of PMSG is similar to -
(a) FSH (b) LH
(c) Progesterone (d) Prostaglandin

117) Which of the following is not a steroid hormone –
(a) Estrogen (b) Progesterone
(c) Prostaglandin (d) Androgen

118) Which of the following is essential for the development of alveolar system of mammary gland –
(a) LH (b) FSH
(c) Estrogen (d) Progesterone

119) Besides corpus luteum, progesterone is also secreted by –
(a) Pituitary gland (b) Thyroid gland
(c) Placenta (d) Uterus

120) Growth of the glandular system of the uterus is caused by –
(a) FSH (b) LH
(c) Estrogen (d) Progesterone

121) For estrous synchronization which of the following hormone is used –
(a) Estrogen (b) Progesterone
(c) LH (d) FSH

122) Luteolytic factor causes –
(a) Formation of the corpus luteum
(b) Regression of corpus luteum
(c) Regression of follicle
(d) All of the above

123) Luteolytic factor acts locally through –
(a) Pituitary- ovarian pathway
(b) Utero-ovarian pathway
(c) Hypothalmo - pituitary pathway
(d) None

124) Proestrual bleeding is observed in –
(a) Bitch (b) Cow
(c) Mare (d) Sheep

125) Post estrual bleeding is observed in –

(a) Cow (b) Mare
(c) Bitch (d) Ewe

126) The number of carucles found in the uterus of cow are –

(a) 25-35 (b) 40-50
(c) 60-70 (d) 80-120

127) The caruncles are found in the uterus of –

(a) Mare (b) Sow
(c) Cow (d) Bitch

128) The atrophy of endometrial glands occur during –

(a) Proestrous (b) Oestrus
(c) Metoestrus (d) Diestrus

129) Cervix is poorly defined in -

(a) Bitch (b) Sow
(c) Cow (d) Sheep

130) FSH is essential for –

(a) Growth of graffian follicle (b) Secretion of estrogen
(c) Both a and b (d) None

131) Excessive and prolong use of estrogen causes –

(a) Abortion in pregnant animals
(b) Nymphomania
(c) Cystic ovary
(d) All of the above

132) Increased migration of the leucocytes into the uterine lumen is caused by –

(a) FSH (b) Estrogen
(c) Progesterone (d) LH

133) Which of the following is used for the treatment of ketosis –

(a) FSH (b) TSH
(c) ACTH (d) LH

134) Estrogen should not be administered by –
(a) Intra muscular (b) Intra venous
(c) Sub cutaneous (d) All of the above

135) Which of the following is used for Cuboni test –
(a) Serum of pregnant mare (b) Milk of pregnant mare
(c) Urine of pregnant mare (d) None

136) Which is a multiparous animal –
(a) Cow (b) Mare
(c) Bitch (d) Goat

137) Trichomonas fetus infection is transmitted by –
(a) Inhalation (b) Coitus
(c) Ingestion (d) All of the above

138) The major symptom of trichomoniasis in bovine is –
(a) Post coital pyometra (b) Short oestrus cycle
(c) Prolonged oestrus cycles (d) All of above

139) Uterus is most sensitive to the infection during –
(a) Follicular phase (b) Luteal phase
(c) Proestrus (d) Oestrus

140) MOET means –
(a) Multiple ovulation and embryo transfer
(b) Many oestrus test
(c) Mal orange embryo transfer
(d) None of the above

141) Cystic ovarian syndrome in bovines is due to –
(a) Hormonal derangement of LH
(b) Deficiency of cholesterol
(c) Hypocalcemia
(d) All of the above

142) Progesterone estimation in cows is mainly useful for
(a) Early pregnancy diagnosis (b) Detection of estrus
(c) Detection of laminitis (d) None of the

143) In adrenal virilism the level of which of the following is increased –

(a) Adrenaline (b) Progesterone

(c) 17-ketosteroids (d) Cortisol

144) Endometrium is the inner most layer of –

(a) Vulva (b) Vagina

(c) Uterus (d) Cervix

145) Split oestrus is common in –

(a) Mare (b) Sheep

(c) Bitches (d) Goat

Obstetrics

146) In case of buffaloes the most common cause of dystocia is -

(a) Primary uterine inertia

(b) Foetal monster

(c) Abnormal presentation, position and posture

(d) Pelvic abnormality

147) In case of pig the type of placental classification -

(a) Diffuse (b) Zonary

(c) Discoid (d) Cotyledomary

148) In mares post partum estrus usually occurs -

(a) 5-15 days after foaling (b) 20-30 days after foaling

(c) 30-40 days after foaling (d) 40-50 days after foaling

149) Greenish lochial discharge is observed in -

(a) Cattle (b) Swine

(c) Canine (d) Mare

150) Pseudo pregnancy may occur as a result of increased concentration of -

(a) FSH (b) LH

(c) Oxytocin (d) Prolactin

151) Lutinizing hormones can be used for the treatment of -

(a) Anovulation (b) Genital prolapse

(c) Anoestrus (d) Pyometra

152) In mares the normal time required for expulsion of foetal membranes is -

(a) 8-12 hrs (b) 6-8 hrs
(c) 3-4 hrs (d) Less than one hour

153) Stimulation of cervix is essential for ovulation in -

(a) Buffalo (b) Mare
(c) Rabbit (d) Cow

154) Anovulatory estrus is more common in -

(a) Swine (b) Sheep
(c) Cattle (d) Bitch

155) In cattle maximum early embryonic mortality occur during -

(a) 5-8 days of gestation (b) 8-16 days of gestation
(c) 16-24 days of gestation (d) 24-32 days of gestation

156) In cows the fetal mummification occurs mainly -

(a) 2-3 months of gestations (b) 3-4 months of gestations
(c) 1-2 months of gestations (d) 5-7 months of gestations

157) Bilateral hip flexion posture is also known as -

(a) Dog sitting (b) Breech presentation
(c) Nape posture (d) None of these

158) In India the most common cause of anoestrus is -

(a) Nutritional deficiency (b) Hormonal Imbalance
(c) Over feeding (d) Genetic causes

159) Transcortin binds -

(a) Estrogen (b) Progesterone
(c) Testosterone (d) Thyroxin

160) In case of sheep incomplete dilation of the cervix is known as -

(a) Uterine inertia (b) Casting of weather
(c) Ring womb (d) Uterine torsion

161) The medium used for uterine flushing should be buffered to maintain a pH of -

(a) 6.2-6.4 (b) 6.5-6.89
(c) 8.2-8.4 (d) 7.2-7.6

162) The osmolarity of uterine flushing medium should be -

(a) 250-260 m OSM/kg (b) 270-310 m OSM/kg
(c) 350-400 m OSM/kg (d) 400-450 m OSM/kg

163) The Rush catheter is used for -

(a) Dilatation of the cervix (b) Intra uterine infusion
(c) Embryo collection (d) None of these

164) In vaginal prolapse cases the epidural administration of 2% xylocaine is recommended -

(a) 20-30 ml (b) 40-50 ml
(c) 6-8 ml (d) 1-2 ml

165) During luteal phase the level of the following is increased -

(a) Cortisol (b) Estradiol
(c) Progesterone (d) Adrenalin

166) Abortion due to Brucellosis occurs in cow during -

(a) 2 months (b) 4 months
(c) 5 months (d) During 3rd trimester

167) Fetotomy is recommended in the following conditions -

(a) Dead fetus (b) Twin pregnancy
(c) Torsion of uterus (d) Abnormal live fetus

168) In dog sitting posture the presentation of fetus is -

(a) Anterior longitudinal (b) Posterior longitudinal
(c) Transverse (d) Oblique

169) Calf hood vaccination is done for -

(a) Theileria (b) IBR
(c) Brucellosis (d) None of these

170) Schistomus reflexus is more common in -

(a) Cow (b) Ewe

(c) Mare (d) Bitch

171) Wry neck posture is more commonly found in

(a) Mare (b) Cow

(c) Ewe (d) Bitch

172) Condition characterized by the birth of dummy or bawlers calves is known -

(a) Hydrocephalus (b) Hydramnion

(c) Hydrallantois (d) None of these

173) Cloud burst is pseudo pregnancy of -

(a) Sow (b) Doe

(c) Cow (d) Mare

174) Uterine prolapse is also known as

(a) Ring womb (b) Uterine torsion

(c) Casting of calfbed (d) None of these

175) Uterine torsion is more common in -

(a) Ewe (b) Mare

(c) Buffalo (d) Bitch

176) Fetal cotyledons and maternal caruncles join to form -

(a) Placenta (b) Placentome

(c) Vestibule (d) Thick membrane

177) Hip flexion posture may lead to -

(a) Death of fetus (b) Oedema of the body

(c) Post partum paralysis (d) None of these

178) The act of parturition in bitches is known as -

(a) Kidding (b) Delivery

(c) Foaling (d) Whelping

179) Winkler's sutures involve the fixation of -
(a) Inner canthus with eyelid
(b) Medial and lateral patellar ligaments
(c) Diaphragm and displaced abomasum
(d) Cervix and prepubic tendon

180) Posterior epidural anesthesia is recommended for -
(a) Caesarean operation (b) Udder surgery
(c) Prolapse of uterus (d) All of these

181) Involution of uterus in buffaloes takes place within -
(a) 10 days (b) 20 days
(c) 30 days (d) 40 days

182) The most common obstetrical disorder in bovine is –
(a) Dystocia
(b) Genital prolapse
(c) Retention of fetal membranes
(d) Uterine torsion

183) Epidosin can be used for the treatment of-
(a) Uterine torsion (b) Genital prolapse
(c) Ring womb (d) None

184) PGF2 alpha can be used for the treatment of –
(a) Uterine prolapse (b) True anestrous
(c) PCL (d) None

185) Waxing of teat is one of the symptoms approaching parturition in –
(a) Swine (b) Mare
(c) Ewe (d) Cow

186) Bang,s disease is also known as –
(a) Vibriosis (b) Brucellosis
(c) Leptspirosis (d) Trichomoniasis

187) Papyraceous mummification is commonaly found in –
(a) Bovine (b) Equine
(c) Canine (d) None

188) Uterine torsion is more common in –
(a) Mare (b) Sheep
(c) Buffalo (d) Bitch

189) Lack of uterine contractions is known as –
(a) Uterine prolapse (b) Uterine torsion
(c) Uterine inertia (d) None

190) Melengesterol acetate is a synthetic –
(a) Oestrogen (b) Progesterone
(c) PGF_2 alpha (d) Gonadotropin

191) In mares foal heat can be observed during –
(a) 5-12 days post partum (b) 20-30 days post partum
(c) 30-40 days post partum (d) 40-50 days post partum

192) The conversion of progesterone into estrogen is stimulated due to rise in –
(a) Fetal adrenalin (b) Fetal cortisol
(c) Fetal nor adrenalin (d) None

193) Lochial discharge is usually ceased by 48 hours post partum in –
(a) Cow (b) Mare
(c) Buffalo (d) Sheep

194) Incomplete dilatation of cervix may be due to –
(a) Hormonal dysfunction (b) Uterine inertia
(c) Dead fetus (d) Uterine torsion

195) The accumulation of water in side the uterus is known as –
(a) Pyometra (b) Mucometra
(c) Hydrometra (d) None

196) In buffaloes the type of placenta is –
(a) Diffuse (b) Cotyledonary
(c) Zonary (d) None

197) The discoid type of placenta is found in –
(a) Sheep (b) Mare
(c) Cow (d) Man

198) The endotheliochorial placenta is found in -

(a) Pig (b) Sheep
(c) Dog (d) Cow

199) The epitheliochorial placenta is found in –

(a) Buffaloes (b) Bitch
(c) Man (d) None

200) In monkey the type of placenta is –

(a) Zonary (b) Diffuse
(c) Cotyledonary (d) Discoid

201) The hemochorial placenta is found in –

(a) Man (b) Pig
(c) Dog (d) None

202) In case of sow the normal duration of 3rd stage of labor is –

(a) 1-4 hours (b) 4-6 hours
(c) 6-8 hours (d) None

203) In case of pregnant mares endometrial cups are formed during-

(a) 1st month of pregnancy
(b) During 2nd month of pregnancy
(c) During 3rd month of pregnancy
(d) During 4th month of pregnancy

204) In case of mares corpus luteum verum can only be palpated per rectum for –

(a) 2-3 days after its formation
(b) 7-8 days after its
(c) 10-12 days after its formation
(d) 15-16 days after its formation

205) The day of definite attachment of conceptus in cow is -

(a) 15-20days (b) 25-30 days
(c) 30-35 days (d) 40-45 days

206) The day of definite attachment of conceptus in sow is –

(a) Day 12 (b) Day 15
(c) Day 18 (d) Day 25

207) The day of definite attachment of conceptus in ewe is –
(a) 12-13 days (b) 15-16 days
(c) 25-30days (d) 30-35 days

208) The day of definite attachment of conceptus in mare is –
(a) 10-12 days (b) 15-20days
(c) 25-38 days (d) 40-45 days

209) The hormonal theory of parturition suggest that the parturition in cattle is initiated by –
(a) Increased fetal production of corticoids
(b) Increased level of progesterone
(c) Decreased Level of estrogen
(d) Decreased level of prostaglandin

210) The hormones responsible for ripening of the cervix are –
(a) Estrogen
(b) Estrogen and relaxin
(c) Estrogen, relaxin and cortisol
(d) Estrogen, relaxin, cortisol and prostaglandin

211) The second and third stage of parturition is interspersed in –
(a) Goat (b) Mare
(c) Cow (d) Bitch

212) The enzyme that convert placentally derived progesterone to estrogen before parturition -
(a) 17 alpha Hydroxylase (b) 17 beta Hydroxylase
(c) Aromatase (d) Phospholipase A2

213) Which of the following is essential for the development of alveolar system of mammary gland –
(a) LH (b) FSH
(c) Estrogen (d) Progesterone

214) Besides corpus luteum, progesterone is also secreted by –
(a) Pituitary gland (b) Thyroid gland
(c) Placenta (d) Uterus

215) Growth of the glandular system of the uterus is caused by –
(a) FSH (b) LH
(c) Estrogen (d) Progesterone

216) The number of carucles found in the uterus of cow are –
(a) 25-35 (b) 40-50
(c) 60-70 (d) 80-120

217) The caruncles are found in the uterus of –
(a) Mare (b) Sow
(c) Cow (d) Bitch

218) The atrophy of endometrial glands occur during –
(a) Proestrous (b) Oestrus
(c) Metoestrus (d) Diestrus

219) Instead of caruncles longitudinal folds are found in the uterus of –
(a) Cow (b) Mare
(c) Buffalo (d) Ewe

220) The placentome is formed by-
(a) Caruncle (b) Chorionic villi
(c) Both a and b (d) None

221) Excessive and prolong use of estrogen causes –
(a) Abortion in pregnant animals
(b) Nymphomania
(c) Cystic ovary
(d) All of the above

222) Loosening of the pubic symphysis is caused by –
(a) Estrogen (b) Progesterone
(c) FSH (d) LH

223) Epiphyseal growth of the bone is caused by –
(a) Estrogen (b) Progesterone
(c) FSH (d) LH

224) Which of the following may cause retention of the fetal membranes in bovines -

(a) Hypocalcemia
(b) Lack of iodine
(c) Lack of selenium
(d) All of the above

225) Hen's egg shaped amniotic vesicle can be observed in cow during -

(a) 30-40 days of gestation
(b) 60-90 days of gestation
(c) 100-120 days of gestation
(d) All of the above

226) Location of pregnant uterus during 5-6 months of pregnancy in cow is -

(a) At pelvic brim
(b) Pelvic cavity
(c) Forward and downward in the abdominal cavity
(d) All of the above

227) Oozing of colustrum before two days of parturition is observed in case of -

(a) Mare
(b) Cow
(c) Bitch
(d) Ewe

228) During pregnancy diagnosis in cows, placentomes can be palpated at -

(a) 30-40 days of gestation
(b) 40-60 days of gestation
(c) 60-70 days of gestation
(d) 100 days and above

229) Which of the following is used for Cuboni test -

(a) Serum of pregnant mare
(b) Milk of pregnant mare
(c) Urine of pregnant mare
(d) None

230) Which is a sign of approaching parturition in cow -

(a) Tenacious white mucus discharge from vulva
(b) Enlargement of mammary gland
(c) 2-6 times enlarged vulva
(d) All of the above

231) After parturition fetal membrane is detached because of -

(a) Reduced blood supply
(b) Caruncle reduce in size
(c) Contraction of uterine musculature
(d) All of the above

232) An additional symptom which is seen in bitch approaching parturition in contrast to cow –

(a) Enlargement of the mammary gland
(b) Oedematous swelling of the vulva
(c) Vulvar Discharge
(d) Panting

233) Expulsion of the fetus occurs during which stage of parturition –

(a) During first stage of parturition
(b) During second stage of parturition
(c) During third Stage of parturition
(d) None

234) Expulsion of dead fetus after completion of full term of gestation is known as –

(a) Abortion (b) Stillbirth
(c) Premature birth (d) None

235) Expulsion of dead fetus before completion of full term of gestation is known as –

(a) Abortion (b) Premature birth
(c) Still birth (d) Normal birth

236) In case of cows which type of fetal mummification is seen –

(a) Hematinic (b) Paperaceous
(c) Both of them (d) None of the above

237) In which condition corpus luteum persists –

(a) Fetal mummification (b) Abortion
(c) Estrus (d) All of the above

238) Hypothalamic hormones are small molecules of –

(a) Arachidonic acid (b) Peptide
(c) Starch (d) None

239) In polytocus animals which type of mummification is commonly observed –

(a) Hematinic (b) Papyraceous type
(c) Both a and b (d) None of the above

240) During right side uterine torsion, rolling of the animal on the earth is done in -

(a) Same direction (b) Opposite direction
(c) Any of the two (d) None of the above

241) The most preferred treatment of uterine torsion is –

(a) Rolling of the dam (b) Caesarean section
(c) Laparotomy (d) None of the above

242) The most common cause of dystocia in bovines is –

(a) Abnormal presentation, position and posture
(b) Disproportion between pelvis and fetus
(c) Pelvic stenosis
(d) None of the above

243) Inter cornual ligament is strong in –

(a) Cow (b) Bitch
(c) Cat (d) All of the above

244) Inter cornual ligament is absent in –

(a) Cow (b) Bitch
(c) Cat (d) Both b and c

245) Endothelial chorial placenta is found in –

(a) Bitch (b) Cat
(c) Deer (d) Both a & b

246) In rabbit, the type of placenta found is –

(a) Diffused (b) Zonary
(c) Discoidal (d) Cotyledonary

247) The amnion is developed from –

(a) Ectoderm (b) Mesoderm
(c) Endoderm (d) None of the above

248) The allantois is developed from –

(a) Endoderm and splanchnopleuric mesoderm
(b) Endoderm and mesoderm
(c) Ectoderm and mesoderm
(d) None of the above

249) In which animal the allantois is attached to amnion-

(a) Cow (b) Pig
(c) Dog (d) Both a and b

250) Schistosomus reflexus is most common in -

(a) Cattle (b) Sheep
(c) Swine (d) All of the above

251) The condition characterized by the birth of dummy or bawler's calf is known as -

(a) Hydrocephalus (b) Epitheliogenesis cogenita
(c) Ichthyosis (d) Hypotrichosis congenital

252) The condition where straight rear legs and contracted gastronemius muscle are formed is known As -

(a) Syndacrylism (b) Spastic paresis
(c) Hydrocephalus (d) Syndactilism

253) Which of the following is the anomaly of the trunk -

(a) Schistosomus reflesus (b) Spastic paresis
(c) Hydrocephalus (d) Syndactilism

254) During handling the dystocia hooks are the instruments used -

(a) Traction (b) Rotation
(c) Repulsion (d) All of the above

255) During handling the case of dystocia which of the following is used for repulsion -

(a) Snares (b) Hooks
(c) Repellor (d) Rope

256) Cruch repellor is used for -

(a) Repulsion (b) Section
(c) Traction (d) All of the above

257) The operation by which the fetus is returned to its normal presentation, position and posture is Known as -

(a) Mutation (b) Rotation
(c) Repulsion (d) None of the above

258) The operation by which the fetus is pushed back from pelvic to abdominal cavity is called as –

(a) Detorsion (b) Rotation
(c) Repulsion (d) Adjustment

259) Turning of fetus on its long axis to bring the fetus into dorso- sacral position is known as –

(a) Rotation (b) Repulsion
(c) Adjustment (d) All of the above

260) Prostaglandin F2 alpha is used for –

(a) Treatment of cystic ovary (b) Fetal mummification
(c) Estrus synchronization (d) All of the

261) In threatened abortion which of the following is used –

(a) Oestrogen (b) Progesterone
(c) PGF_2 alpha (d) All of the above

262) For let down of milk most common drug used is –

(a) Oestrogen (b) Progesterone
(c) PGF_2 alpha (d) Oxytocin

263) Site of fertilization in mammals is –

(a) Cervix (b) Uterus
(c) Ovary (d) Fallopian tube

264) Which of the following is a induced ovulator –

(a) Cow (b) Bitch
(c) Cat (d) Camel

265) Stimulation of cervix is essential for ovulation in –

(a) Cows (b) Buffalo
(c) Mare (d) Camel

266) In buffaloes the average gestation period is –

(a) 290 days (b) 310 days
(c) 330 days (d) 360 days

267) In bitches the average gestation period is -
(a) 62 days (b) 70 days
(c) 80 days (d) 100 days

268) Non Sexual erection of penis is known as -
(a) Pederasty (b) Priapism
(c) Carnal intercourse (d) Satyiasis

269) Buhner's technique is used for the treatment of -
(a) Genital prolapse (b) Uterine torsion
(c) Ring womb (d) Cystic ovarian degeneration

270) The time of ovulation in case of cow is -
(a) During early estrus (b) During middle estrus
(c) During late estrous (d) After end of estrus

271) The time of ovulation in case of mare is
(a) Early estrus (b) Middle estrus
(c) Late estrus (d) After end of estrus

272) The time of ovulation in case of ewe is -
(a) Early estrus (b) Middle estrus
(c) Late estrus (d) End of estrus

273) The time of ovulation in case of bitch is -
(a) Early estrus (b) Middle estrus
(c) Late estrus (d) After end of estrus

274) The time of ovulation in case of cat is -
(a) Early estrus (b) Middle estrus
(c) 24-30 hours after coitus (d) Late estrus

Andrology

275) In bull fetus primordial germ cell migrate to the gonadal ridge, about day -
(a) 26 (b) 50
(c) 75 (d) 80

276) Adrogens are produced by -
(a) Lutein cells (b) Leydig cells
(c) Sertoli cells (d) Theca interna cells

277) The maximum concentration of ergothionine is found in the semen of -
(a) Bull (b) Ram
(c) Stallion (d) Dog

278) The sperm concentration in boar semen is -
(a) 800-2000 million/ml (b) 2000-3000 million/ml
(c) 200-300 million/ml (d) 1000-1500 million/ml

279) The major site for sperm capacitation appear to be the -
(a) Vagina (b) Cervix
(c) Uterus (d) Oviduct

280) During courtship Estrus grunts are common in -
(a) Cattle (b) Sheep
(c) Goat (d) Swine

281) The semen samples should be discarded if the sperm concentration in bulls is less than -
(a) 500 million/ml (b) 700 million/ml
(c) 800 million/ml (d) 700 million/ml

282) Fibrosis and calcification of testis is observed in which of the following
(a) Testicular Hypoplasia (b) Testicular Degeneration
(c) Testicular Tumors (d) Orchitis

283) Maturation and storage of spermatozoa occur in -
(a) Testes (b) Epididymes
(c) Seminal vesicle (d) Vas deference

284) The first attempt for semen collection by electro - ejaculation method was attempted by -
(a) Case (b) Baltelk
(c) Gunn (d) Ivan off

285) The Danish model of AV is about -

(a) 16″ x 2.5″ (b) 24″ x 2.2″
(c) 12″x 3″ (d) 28″x 3.5″

286) The secondary sperm abnormalities are due to dysfunction of -

(a) Testes (b) Epididymes
(c) Vas deferens (d) Urethra

287) The tertiary abnormalities are due to

(a) Dysfunction of scrotum (b) Dysfunction of testes
(c) Dysfunction of epididymes (d) Mishandling of semen

288) The sperm abnormalities have been classified as major and minor sperm defects by

(a) Erick Bloom (b) Roberts
(c) Foote (d) Hafez

289) Pouch formation by invagination of the nuclear membrane is seen in -

(a) Dag defect (b) Diadem defect
(c) Knobbed sperm defect (d) Decapitated sperm defect

290) The Dag defect seems to occur during the passage through the -

(a) Urethra (b) Caput epididymes
(c) Cauda epididymes (d) Testes

291) In MBRT, a good quality semen would reduce the methylene blue in only -

(a) 3-5 minutes (b) 5-10 minutes
(c) 10-15 minutes (d) 15-20 minutes

292) High percentage of abnormal sperms is termed as -

(a) Necrozoo spermia (b) Teratozoo spermia
(c) Azoospermia (d) Oligospermia

293) Coconut milk extender was evolved by -

(a) Norman *et al.* (b) Forte *et al.*
(c) Salisburry *et al.* (d) Norman *et al.*

294) The most commonly used dilutor for preservation of bull semen is-
(a) EYP (b) EYC
(c) IVT (d) CUE

295) The surface area of French medium straw is -
(a) 555 mm (b) 825 mm
(c) 950 mm (d) 1152 mm

296) In boar sperm cell contribute on an average -
(a) 15% of the semen by volume
(b) 10% of the semen by volume
(c) 8% of the semen by volume
(d) 2-5% of the semen by volume

297) Fructose is absent in the semen of -
(a) Stallion (b) Boar
(c) Ram (d) Dog

298) During AI with frozen semen the most appropriate site of semen deposition is -
(a) Anterior vagina (b) Mid Cervix
(c) Anterior cervix (d) Uterine horn

299) The blood supply to the testes is by -
(a) Internal iliac artery (b) Pudic artery
(c) Spermatic artery (d) External pudic artery

300) The OS penis is found in -
(a) Stallian (b) Dog
(c) Ram (d) Boar

301) The terminal pert of penis contains several spines in -
(a) Dog (b) Ram
(c) Cat (d) Boar

302) The urethral process is present in the penis of -
(a) Ram (b) Dog
(c) Boar (d) Stallion

303) During deep freezing the level of glycerol should be

(a) 5% (b) 7%

(c) 10% (d) 15%

304) In case of cattle the testicles descend from abdomen to the scrotum at -

(a) 3.5 -4 months months of gestation

(b) 5-6 months of gestation

(c) 6-7 months of gestation

(d) 7-8 months of gestation

305) In case of stallion the testicles are descended from abdomen to the scrotum at-

(a) 2-3 months of gestation (b) 3-4 months of gestation

(c) 5-7 months of gestation (d) 9-11 months of gestation

306) In case of pig the testicles descend from abdomen to the scrotum at-

(a) 1-2 months of gestation (b) 70 days of gestation

(c) 90 days of gestation (d) None

307) In case of dog the testicles descend from abdomen to the scrotum at -

(a) 20 days of gestation (b) 30 days of gestation

(c) 40 days of gestation (d) 5 days after birth

308) The total length of seminiferous tubules in bull is -

(a) 300 meters (b) 1000 meters

(c) 3000 meters (d) 5000 meters

309) In case of dog the total length of seminiferous tubules is -

(a) 50 meters (b) 100 meters

(c) 150 meters (d) 200 meters

310) The blood testes permeability barrier is formed by –

(a) Leydig cells (b) Sertoli cells

(c) Germinal epithelial cells (d) None

311) The total length of epididymes in bull is -

(a) 10 meters (b) 20 meters
(c) 30 meters (d) 40 meters

312) The total length of epididymes in stallion is -

(a) 20 meters (b) 30 meters
(c) 40 meters (d) 50 meters

313) The total length of epididymes in boar is-

(a) 20 meters (b) 50 meters
(c) 80 meters (d) 100 meters

314) The total duration of epididymal journey of spermatozoa in bull is-

(a) 10 days (b) 20 days
(c) 30 days (d) 50 days

315) The total duration of epididymal journey of spermatozoa in boar is-

(a) 5-7 days (b) 7-9 days
(c) 9-12 days (d) 15-20 days

316) The fossa glandis is found in the glans penis of -

(a) Bull (b) Stallion
(c) Boar (d) Ram

317) The post scrotal sigmoid flexure is found in the penis of -

(a) Bull (b) Ram
(c) Boar (d) Stallion

318) The pre scrotal sigmoid flexure is found in the penis of -

(a) Stallion (b) Bull
(c) Ram (d) Boar

319) The cork screw type penis is found -

(a) Ram (b) Bull
(c) Stallion (d) Boar

320) Os penis is found in -

(a) Boar (b) Dog
(c) Stallion (d) Ram

321) Courtship bleats are observed during sexual play in -

(a) Bull (b) Ram
(c) Stallion (d) Boar

322) Nudging of the female through forelegs is commonly seen in -

(a) Cattle (b) Sheep and goat
(c) Swine (d) Equine

323) During sexual play male bites over the females body in case of -

(a) Stallion (b) Ram
(c) Bull (d) Boar

324) The first scientific work in A.I. in dogs was performed by -

(a) Roberts (b) Lazzaro Spallanzani
(c) Zemjanis (d) Hafez

325) In India artificial insemination was introduced by -

(a) Madan (b) P. Bhattarcharya
(c) Sampat Kumaran (d) None

326) Semen collection in bull by massage method was reported by -

(a) Case (b) Roberts
(c) Zemjamis (d) None

327) The first attempt for semen collection by electro-ejaculation was attempted in 1922 by -

(a) Case (b) Nakao
(c) Baltelli (d) None

328) The first A.V. for bulls was designed by -

(a) Tomar (b) Bhosrekar
(c) Komorou (d) None

329) The water content in the semen ranged from -

(a) 50-60% (b) 60-70%
(c) 70-80% (d) 85-98%

330) The sperm cell contribute on an average by volume in bull -

(a) 3-5% (b) 5-7%
(c) 10% (d) None

331) The sperm cell contribute on an average by volume in boar -

(a) 2-5% (b) 5-10%
(c) 10-12% (d) 15-20%

332) The contribution of secretions from vesicular glands is -

(a) 20-30% (b) 31-38%
(c) 40-50% (d) 50-60%

333) The contribution of secretions from epididymes is -

(a) 10-15% (b) 20-25%
(c) 31-36% (d) 40-50%

334) The contribution of secretions from Prostate and Bulbo urethral glands is -

(a) 5-10% (b) 10-20%
(c) 20-25% (d) 31-32%

335) In ruminants the normal sugar providing energy to the spermatozoa is -

(a) Dextrose (b) Fructose
(c) Glucose (d) Manose

336) The average level of Fructose in the semen of bull is

(a) 100 mg/100 ml (b) 200 mg/100 ml
(c) 400 mg/100 ml (d) 500 mg/100 ml

337) The fertile life of spermatozoa in the genital tract of cow is –

(a) 10-15 hours (b) 20-25 hours
(c) 30-48 hours (d) 50-60 hours

338) In the uterus the seminal plasma has -
(a) Immunosuppressive effect (b) Antimicrobial effect
(c) Antiseptic effect (d) None

339) The fertile life of spermatozoa in the female genital tract of mare is–
(a) 10-20 hours (b) 20-30 hours
(c) 40-50 hours (d) 72-120 hours

340) The fertile life of spermatozoa in the female genital tract of ewe is -
(a) 10-15 hours (b) 15- 25 hours
(c) 30-48 hours (d) 50-60 hours

341) The fertile life of spermatozoa in the female genital tract of sow is
(a) 15-20 hrs (b) 5-10 hours
(c) 24-72 hours (d) 80-100 hours

342) During courtship mock fighting is being observed in -
(a) Cattle (b) Equine
(c) Canine (d) Swine

343) Optimum time for service in sow is -
(a) 5-10 hours after the onset of estrum
(b) 12-30 hours after the onset of estrum
(c) 36-48 hours after the onset of estrum
(d) 50-70 hours after the onset of estrum

344) The optimum time of service in bitch is -
(a) 1-2 days after the onset of estrum
(b) 4-6 days after the onset of estrum
(c) 1-2 days after the end of estrum
(d) 4-6 days after the end of estrum

345) The normal average sperm concentration in bull should be -
(a) 500 million per ml (b) 700 million per ml
(c) 1000 million per ml (d) 1500 million per ml

346) In buffalo bull the normal sperm concentration should be -
(a) 300 million per ml (b) 600 million per ml
(c) 900 million per ml (d) 1400 million per ml

347) In stallion the normal sperm concentration should be –
(a) 200million per ml (b) 400 million per ml
(c) 700 million per ml (d) 1000 million per ml

348) In ram the normal sperm concentration should be
(a) 500 million per ml (b) 1000 million per ml
(c) 1500 million per ml (d) 2000 million per ml

349) The normal sperm concentration in boar should be –
(a) 100 million per ml (b) 300 million per ml
(c) 500 million per ml (d) 700 million per ml

350) The normal sperm concentration in dog should be –
(a) 300 million per ml (b) 500 million per ml
(c) 700 million per ml (d) 1200 million per ml

351) In man the normal sperm concentration should be –
(a) 150 million per ml (b) 600 million per ml
(c) 800 million per ml (d) 1200 million per ml

352) The age at puberty in cross-bred bulls is –
(a) 5-10 months (b) 12-18 months
(c) 20-30 months (d) 30-40 months

353) The age at puberty in buffalo bull is –
(a) 6-10 months (b) 12-18 months
(c) 24-30 months (d) 36-48 months

354) The age at puberty in stallion is –
(a) 8-12 months (b) 18-24 months
(c) 30-36 months (d) 36-48 months

355) The age at puberty in ram is –
(a) 7-8 months (b) 12-18 months
(c) 20-24 months (d) 24-30 months

356) The age at puberty in boar is –
(a) 6-7 months (b) 10-15 months
(c) 18-24 months (d) 24-30 months

357) The age at puberty in dog is –

(a) 8-10 months (b) 12-18 months
(c) 18-24 months (d) 24-36 months

358) Most of the inseminations before the advent of frozen semen were performed with semen stored at-

(a) 0 degree centigrade (b) 5 degree centigrade
(c) 10 degree centigrade (d) 20 degree centigrade

359) When the semen is frozen spermatozoa may remain fertile for –

(a) 1 year (b) 2 year
(c) 3 year (d) Indefinite

360) The seminal plasma has an osmotic pressure of about –

(a) 125 milliosmols (b) 200 milliosmols
(c) 285 milliosmols (d) 500 milliosmols

361) Bull sperm motility and fertility in egg yolk is maintained at near –

(a) Acidic pH (b) Alkaline pH
(c) Neutral pH (d) All of the above

362) The most effective means of protecting spermatozoa against the effect of chilling is to provide them-

(a) Lecithin (b) Proteins
(c) Lipoproteins (d) All of the above

363) The first media used to dilute semen were primarily –

(a) Egg yolk (b) Coconut milk
(c) Triss (d) Salt and sugar solution

364) Which part of the female genital tract acts as reservoir for spermatozoa –

(a) Vagina (b) Cervix
(c) Body of uterus (d) Oviduct

365) The first calf following AI with frozen semen was reported in the year –

(a) 1947 (b) 1951
(c) 1960 (d) 1965

366) The initial successful attempt for freezing of spermatozoa at -79 celsius was reported by-

(a) Polge (b) Roberts
(c) Hafez (d) Rowson

367) The commonly used model of AV for collection of bull semen is –

(a) Russian (b) Danish
(c) Swedish (d) Japanese

368) The most critical temperature for spermatozoa during freezing and thawing is between –

(a) 5-10°C (b) 10-15°C
(c) -15 to -60°C (d) None

369) The cellular damage to spermatozoa during freezing occurs due to–

(a) Internal ice crystal formation
(b) Increased solute concentration
(c) Both a and b
(d) None

370) The spermicidal factor present in milk is –

(a) Lectenin (b) Laithin
(c) Lactose (d) Fructose

371) At what temperature time protocol should milk be heated to destroy the spermicidal factor present in it before being used for extending semen –

(a) Boiled for 5 minutes (b) 92-95°C for 10 minutes
(c) 60-65°C for 10 minutes (d) 70-80°C

372) Zwitter-ionic buffers are being preferred for extending the semen because they –

(a) Are easily available
(b) Have better buffering capacity
(c) Easy microscopic examination of extended semen
(d) Prevent cellular damage during freezing

373) Teasing of breeding bulls before semen collection may result in –
(a) Increased semen volume
(b) Increased semen volume as well as increased sperm concentration
(c) Reduced semen volume and sperm concentration
(d) No effect

374) The equilibration time needed for freezing of bull spermatozoa is –
(a) 4 hours at room temperature
(b) 4 hours at 5°C
(c) 6 hours at 20°C
(d) 10 hours at 10°C

375) Small ejaculate volume may be because of –
(a) Incomplete ejaculation (b) Excessive use of bulls
(c) Seminal vesiculitis (d) All of the above

376) The viral contamination of the frozen semen which renders it unfit for A.I.is –
(a) Bovine viral diarrhoea virus
(b) Bovine herpes virus
(c) Blue tongue virus
(d) All of the above

377) The semen from the ram can be collected more frequently because they have –
(a) Short spermatogenic cycle
(b) Higher sperm production rate
(c) Large epididymal sperm reserve
(d) All of the above

378) The site of AI with frozen stallion semen is –
(a) Intra uterine (b) Intra cervical
(c) Anterior Vagina (d) All of the above

379) In which of the following species AI was tried –
(a) Bovine (b) Caprine
(c) Canine (d) Equine

380) Which of the following is not added in the frozen semen because of its toxicity –

(a) Penicillin (b) Streptomycin
(c) Chloramphenicol (d) Sulfonamide

381) The use of insulating bag is done to prevent –

(a) Spilling of semen
(b) Trickling of water into the collection tube
(c) Sunlight
(d) Contamination shock

382) The first method of semen collection used was –

(a) Swab method (b) Fistula method
(c) AV method (d) Massage method

383) By increased frequency of semen collection there will be –

(a) Adverse effect on the quality of semen
(b) Increased microbial load
(c) Change in color
(d) None

384) The detailed structure of the spermatozoa was first studied by –

(a) L. Spallanzani (b) AV Lewenhock
(c) E.I. Evanhoff (d) Roberts

385) The addition of glycerol to the dilutor preserves the integrity of the sperm head by

(a) Providing metabolic substrates
(b) Creating intracellular equilibration
(c) The action of Dessication
(d) None

386) The yellow color of the Jersey bull semen may be because of -

(a) Riboflavin (b) Cynocobalamine
(c) Provitamin A (d) None

387) The Dag defect of spermatozoa is grouped under –

(a) Primary abnormalities (b) Secondary abnormalities
(c) Miscellaneous abnormalities (d) None

388) The length of AV cylinder used for semen collection in case of bulls is –

(a) 10 cm (b) 20 cm
(c) 30-40 cm (d) 50-60 cm

389) In AV for the length of inner sleeve is –

(a) 10 cm (b) 20 cm
(c) 30-40 cm (d) 50-55 cm

390) The length of cone used in AV for bulls is –

(a) 7-8 cm (b) 20-25 cm
(c) 25-30 cm (d) 30-35 cm

391) The main objective of dilution of semen is –

(a) To increase the volume of semen
(b) To preserve the fertility of sperm
(c) Both a and b
(d) None of the above

392) The rate of dilution of ram semen is –

(a) 1:4 (b) 1:2
(c) 1:9 (d) 1:105

393) Prostaglandin F2 alpha causes luteolysis of corpus luteum in cows during –

(a) 1-3 days of cycle (b) 3-5 days of cycle
(c) 5-16 days of cycle (d) None

394) The post sperm fraction which is gelatinous is secreted in boar –

(a) Seminal vesicle (b) Prostate
(c) Epididymis (d) Bulbourethral gland

395) Ejaculation occur by digital pressure in case of –

(a) Bull (b) Ram
(c) Stallion (d) Boar

396) Air pump is used in AV of –

(a) Stallion (b) Bull
(c) Boar (d) Ram

397) Semen collection is usually done in stallion by–

(a) Massage Method (b) Recto-ejaculation
(c) AV Method (d) All

398) Recommended dilutor for semen of stallion is –

(a) EYC dilutor (b) Yolk glucose bicarbonate
(c) Glucose gelatin (d) Yolk glucose citrate

399) How many parts of egg yolk is used in sodium citrate dilutors –

(a) 20 (b) 30
(c) 50 (d) 70

400) During AI, the site of semen deposition in mare is –

(a) Cervix (b) Vagina
(c) Uterus (d) All of the above

401) Dose of liquid semen used for AI in cows is –

(a) 1 ml (b) 5 ml
(c) 0.5 ml (d) 0.2 ml

402) Dose of semen as represented by concentration should be in mare–

(a) 15 million/dose (b) 20 million/dose
(c) 50 million /dose (d) 250 million / dose

403) Most important spermicidal heavy metals is -

(a) Cu & Fe (b) Zn
(c) Cd (d) Hg

404) Which cells are more common in severe testicular hypoplasia –

(a) Medusa Cells (b) Giant Cells
(c) Germ Cells (d) Both a & b

405) Glyceryl - Phosphoryl Choline are secreted from

(a) Seminal Vesicle gland (b) Prostate gland
(c) Epididymis (d) Cowper's gland

406) Conception percentage on first insemination in case of cows is –

(a) 70 percent (b) 65 percent
(c) 90 percent (d) 95 percent

407) The first AI in India was performed at -
(a) NDRI Karnal (b) IVRI
(c) Palace dairy farm Mysore (d) NDRI Bangalore

408) Which of the following is the most fragile part of the spermatozoa -
(a) Head (b) Neck
(c) Middle piece (d) Tail

409) Arrangement of fibrils in middle piece of spermatozoa is -
(a) 9+2 (b) 9+2+2
(c) 9+9+2 (d) 11+2

410) Arrangement of fibrils in the tail of spermatozoa is
(a) 9+2 (b) 9+2+2
(c) 9+9+2 (d) 11+2

411) Total length of sperm in bull, ram or boar is -
(a) 66 micron in bull, 68 micron in ram and boar
(b) 68 micron in bull 66 micron in ram and Boar
(c) 66 micron in all
(d) 68 micron in all

412) Which of the following is known as Jensen ring -
(a) Proximal centriole (b) Ring centriole
(c) Broad helix (d) Neck piece

413) The nature of prostatic secretion is -
(a) Acidic (b) Alkaline
(c) Neutral (d) All of the above

414) Optimum temperature for preservation of boar semen in liquid stage is -
(a) 5-10°C (b) 15-18°C
(c) 25-30°C (d) None

415) Which of the following is present in the seminal vesicle secretion of stallion -
(a) Ergothionine (b) Inositol
(c) Citrate (d) Zinc

416) Inositol present in the seminal vesicle secretion of which animal -

(a) Boar (b) Bull
(c) Ram (d) Stallion

417) Which of the following is present in the epididymal secretion in Stallion -

(a) Sorbitol (b) Glycerophosphocholine
(c) Inositol (d) Ergothionine

418) Source of energy for sperm in the female genital tract is -

(a) Glucose (b) Fructose
(c) GPC (d) Ergothionine

419) High Catalase acitivity, reduced fructose and high Ph in semen are indication for–

(a) Testicular hypoplasia (b) Testicular degeneration
(c) Orchitis (d) Seminal Vasiculitis

420) Temperature of AV for bull should be -

(a) 45-50°C (b) 30-45°C
(c) 42-45°C (d) 20-25°C

421) The first AV was prepared by -

(a) Robert (b) Heap
(c) G. Amenta (d) None of the above

422) Fructose for sperm motility is provided by -

(a) Prostate gland (b) Seminal vesicle
(c) Cowpers gland (d) All of the above

423) Outer most layer of the testes is -

(a) Tunica vaginalis (b) Tunica vesculosa
(c) Tunica germina (d) None of the above

424) Mesorchium is -

(a) Peritoneal fold that holds the fetal testes in place
(b) Peritoneal fold that holds the fetal ovary in place
(c) Peritoneal fold that holds the fetal uterus in place
(d) Peritoneal fold that holds the fetal epididymis in place

425) Epididymis originates from -

(a) Wolffian duct (b) Mullerian duct
(c) Para mesonefric duct (d) None of the above

426) Spermatogenesis is mainly under the regulatory influence of -

(a) FSH (b) LH
(c) Parathyroid hormone (d) Testosterone

427) Cryopreservation of the semen was first attempted by -

(a) Parkes (b) Roberts
(c) Hafez (d) Polge

428) Glycerol as a cryoprotectant was discovered by -

(a) Polge (b) Smith
(c) Salisbury (d) Roberts

429) Glycerol as a cryoprotectant was discovered in the year -

(a) 1940 (b) 1945
(c) 1949 (d) 1951

430) Unfertilized ovum remains for months in the oviduct of – –species

(a) Sow (b) Mare
(c) Ewe and Doe (d) Bitch

431) Non Hormonal method of synchronization in ewes -

(a) Flushing (b) Weaning
(c) Artificial light (d) Pheromones

432) Attachment of sperm to the ovum occurs initially at – – –segment of sperm head

(a) Apical (b) Post-acrosomal
(c) Principal (d) Equitoria

433) Diffuse arm like structure of microtubules in the sperm tail are made of proteins

(a) Flactin (b) Tubulin
(c) Spermosin (d) Dynein

434) In boars, seminal vesicles produces – – – – – which acts as chief osmotic pressure regulator in the semen

(a) Ergothionine (b) Citrate
(c) Inositol (d) Fructose

435) Irregular long estrous cycles are mainly due to -

(a) Early Embryonic Mortality (b) Fetal Maceration
(c) Fetal Mummification (d) All of the above

436) The optimum level of glycerol used for deep freezing of bovine spermatozoa should be –

(a) 5 percent (b) 7 percent
(c) 10 percent (d) 14 percent

437) The smallest size of sperm head is found in –

(a) Bull (b) Stallion
(c) Dog (d) Ram

438) The largest size of sperm head is found in –

(a) Stallion (b) Dog
(c) Bull (d) Boar

439) The animal in which the testes descend into the inguinal canal but not into the scrotum is called –

(a) Cryptorchid (b) High flanker
(c) Hypoplastic testes (d) None

440) Water content in semen ranges from –

(a) 50-60 percent (b) 60-70 percent
(c) 70-80 percent (d) 80-90 percent

441) Sertoli cell tumor produce excessive amount of –

(a) Estrogen (b) Progesterone
(c) Testosterone (d) Inhibin

442) The vesicular gland of stallion is -
(a) Kidney shaped (b) Lobulated
(c) Pear shaped (d) Horse shoe shaped

443) The sorbitol is absent in the semen of -
(a) Bull (b) Ram
(c) Buffalo bull (d) Dog

444) Inability of penis to withdraw back into the prepuce–
(a) Phimosis (b) Paraphimosis
(c) Stenosis (d) Strangulation

445) Flehmans reaction is feature of sexual behavior in -
(a) Bull (b) Dog
(c) Boar (d) Ram

446) Ventral deviation of the penis is known as-
(a) Frenulum (b) Phimosis
(c) Rainbow deviation (d) Phalocampsis

447) Fructose is absent in the semen of -
(a) Bull (b) Ram
(c) Goat (d) Dog

448) Tunica dortose muscle is found in -
(a) Penis (b) Prepuce
(c) Scrotum (d) None

449) The inositol present in boar semen is -
(a) Spermicidal (b) Osmotic pressure regulator
(c) Antimicrobial (d) Antibiotic

450) How many spermatids are formed from 10 secondary spermatocytes–
(a) 5 (b) 10
(c) 20 (d) 40

451) Mock fighting is the feature of sexual behavior in -
(a) Boar (b) Bull
(c) Stallion (d) Dog

452) The epidydimes is longest in –

(a) Bull (b) Stallion
(c) Dog (d) Boar

453) Fibro-elastic type of penis is found in –

(a) Bull (b) Stallion
(c) Man (d) Dog

454) Musculo-membranous type of penis is found in –

(a) Stallion (b) Ram
(c) Bull (d) Goat

455) The secretion of seminal vesicle is yellowish in color in –

(a) Stallion (b) Bull
(c) Dog (d) Cat

456) Large amount of erectile tissues are found in the penis of –

(a) Bull (b) Buck
(c) Ram (d) Stallion

457) The cranial portion of the penis is spirally twisted counter clock wise in case of –

(a) Stallion (b) Boar
(c) Bull (d) Dog

458) Fresh bull semen should not be used for freezing if progressive motility is less than

(a) 70 percent (b) 30 percent
(c) 50 percent (d) 60 percent

459) Frozen bull semen should not be used for AI if motility is less than–

(a) 20 percent (b) 50 percent
(c) 30 percent (d) 40 percent

460) Neat semen samples should not be used for AI if the live sperm cells are less than

(a) 20 percent (b) 70 percent
(c) 30 percent (d) 50 percent

461) Frozen thawed semen samples should not be used for AI if live sperm cells are less than -

(a) 55 percent (b) 25 percent
(c) 35 percent (d) 45 percent

462) The frozen semen doses should ideally contain approximately -

(a) 10 million motile sperms (b) 20 million motile sperms
(c) 30 million motile sperms (d) 40 million motile sperms

463) The sperm concentration is maximum in -

(a) Bull (b) Ram
(c) Poultry (d) Dog

464) The sperm concentration is minimum in -

(a) Stallion (b) Boar
(c) Bull (d) Man

465) The per ml sperm concentration in dog semen is -

(a) 500-600 million (b) 100-250 million
(c) 300-400 million (d) 400-500 million

466) The optimum time of insemination in case of cow is -

(a) Early estrous (b) Middle estrous
(c) Late estrous (d) After end of estrous

467) The optimum time of insemination in case of buffalo is -

(a) Early estrous (b) Middle estrous
(c) Late estrous (d) After end of estrous

468) Fertile life span of stallion spermatozoa

(a) 70-120 hours (b) 24-36 hrs
(c) 36-48 hrs (d) 48 hsr

469) The optimum time of insemination in case of bitch is -

(a) Early estrous (b) Middle estrous
(c) Late estrous (d) After end of estrous

470) The optimum time of insemination in case of ewe is –
(a) Early estrous (b) Middle estrous
(c) Late estrous (d) After end of estrous

471) The optimum time of insemination in case of sow is –
(a) Early estrous (b) Middle estrous
(c) Late estrous (d) After end of estrous

472) The optimum time of insemination incase of goat is –
(a) Early estrous (b) Middle estrous
(c) Late estrous (d) After end of estrous

Common Questions

473) For the first time the spermatozoa was observed under the microscope by –
(a) Lazzaro Spallanzani (b) Ivanoff
(c) Leeuwenhock (d) Roberts

474) The first embryo transfer was performed in rabbit in the year –
(a) 1650 (b) 1890
(c) 1950 (d) 2000

475) The first embryo transfer was performed by –
(a) Polge (b) Smith
(c) Walter Heape (d) Roberts

476) T shaped uterus is found in –
(a) Mare (b) Cow
(c) Bitch (d) Sow

477) The largest size of the uterine horn is found in –
(a) Buffalo (b) Cow
(c) Mare (d) Sow

478) The largest size of clitoris is observed in –
(a) Mare (b) Cow
(c) Bitch (d) Sow

479) Removal of uterus is called as -

(a) Castration (b) Prostatectomy
(c) Tuberectomy (d) Hysterectomy

480) Amniocentesis is the process to determine -

(a) Disease of the brain
(b) Disease of the heart
(c) Hereditary disease of the embryo
(d) None

481) Oral contraceptive pills act by -

(a) Forming barrier between sperm and ova
(b) Killing sperm and ova
(c) Killing sperm
(d) Killing ova

482) The cross of a hybrid with to one of the parental type is known as-

(a) Interse mating (b) Out cross
(c) Back cross (d) None of the above

483) Failure of the testes to descend down into scrotum is -

(a) Impotency (b) Vesectomy
(c) Cryptorchidism (d) None of the above

484) In adrenal virilism the level of which of the following is increased -

(a) Adrenaline (b) Progesterone
(c) 17-ketosteroids (d) Cortisol

485) Feminization in dogs is observed in -

(a) Sertoli cell tumor (b) Leydig cell tumor
(c) Klinefelter syndrome (d) All of the above

486) Yolk sac placenta is functional in cow up to -

(a) 100 days (b) 190 days
(c) Very few days (d) 220 days

487) For let down of milk most common drug used is -

(a) Oestrogen (b) Progesterone
(c) PGF2 alpha (d) Oxytocin

488) PgF2á has local effect on ovary in all species except-
(a) Cow (b) Bitch
(c) Mare (d) Sow

489) First successful transfer of fertilized egg was done at –
(a) USA (b) USSR
(c) UK (d) None of the above

490) In India first embryo transfer calf was born at –
(a) NDRI (b) NRCC
(c) NII (d) IVRI

491) First surgical buffalo embryo transfer calf born in Asia at –
(a) NRCC (b) NII
(c) NDRI (d) SAG

492) First non surgical buffalo embryo transfer calf born on –
(a) 4 October 1988 (b) 22nd Dec 1987
(c) 19 March 1988 (d) 16 October 1987

493) Photoperiodism is a characteristic of the sexual activity in –
(a) Sheep, goat and horse (b) Dog
(c) Cow (d) Sow

494) When the semen is frozen spermatozoa may remain fertile for –
(a) 1 year (b) 2 year
(c) 3 year (d) Indefinite

495) The seminal plasma has an osmotic pressure of about –
(a) 125 milliosmols (b) 200 milliosmols
(c) 285 milliosmols (d) 500 milliosmols

496) Bull sperm motility and fertility in egg yolk is maintained at near –
(a) Acidic pH (b) Alkaline pH
(c) Neutral pH (d) All of the above

497) The most effective means of protecting spermatozoa against the effect of chilling is to provide them-
(a) Lecithin (b) Proteins
(c) Lipoproteins (d) All of the above

498) Complete lack of libido is observed–

(a) Testicular hypoplasia (b) Testicular degeneration
(c) Bilateral cryptorchidism (d) Bilateral testicular aplasia

499) The patent ductus arteriosis is more commonly observed in –

(a) Dogs (b) Cattle
(c) Horse (d) Sheep

500) Wrinkler's sutures involve the fixation of -

(a) Inner canthus with eyelid
(b) Medial and lateral patellar ligaments
(c) Diaphragm and displaced abomasum
(d) Cervix and prepubic tendon

501) Centric type of nidation or implantation occurs in

(a) Rodents (b) Primates
(c) Ruminants (d) None of the above

502) Endometrial cups are formed from

(a) Chorionic girdle (fetal origin)
(b) Maternal caruncles
(c) Endometrium (maternal origin)
(d) None of the above

503) In sow, the villi near the endometrial glands are enlarged and specialized to form structures called

(a) Hippomanes (b) Amniotic plaques
(c) Areolae (d) Placentomes

504) Most of the developmental anomalies occur during

(a) Period of embryo (b) Period of ovum
(c) Period of fetus (d) During birth

505) Low land abortion or Marsh land abortion is due to

(a) Fescue poisoning (b) Leptospirosis
(c) Nitrate poisoning (d) None of the above

506) Collaginase used for treatment of Retention of fetal membrane is administered through -

(a) Intra Muscular route (b) Intra Venous route
(c) Intra uterine (d) Retained umbilical cord

507) Mediastinum testis is absent in which of the fowlling

(a) Stallion (b) Post-acrosomal
(c) Principal (d) Equitorial

508) Unique species in which epididymis can produce testosterone

(a) Boar (b) Dog
(c) Bull (d) Stallion

509) Maintenance of CL and Progesterone from CL are necessary throughout the gestation in

(a) Mare (b) Sow
(c) Bitch (d) Cow

510) pH of TRIS extender is

(a) Slightly acidic (b) Slightly alkaline
(c) Neutral (d) Alkaline

511) The first cloned lamb Dolly was produced in the year -

(a) 1980 (b) 1985
(c) 1990 (d) 1996

512) The first time the term nuclear transplantation was proposed by -

(a) Heape (b) John Gurd on
(c) Hans sperman (d) Robert

513) In India first buffalo calf through embryo transfer was reported by-

(a) Talwar *et al.* (b) Madan *et al.*
(c) Mushvg *et al.* (d) Janwar *et al.*

514) In India artificial insemination was introduced by -

(a) P. Bhattacharya (b) Kumaran
(c) Perry (d) None of the above

515) Potato soup pyometra or post service pyometra is characteristic of – – – – – – –infection–

(a) Trichomoniasis (b) Vibriosis
(c) Brucellosis (d) All

516) The most common cause of orchitis in bulls–

(a) Leptospirosis (b) Brucellosis
(c) Trichomoniasis (d) Vibriosis

517) Urethral process is present in the penis–

(a) Dog & Buck (b) Buck & Stallion
(c) Stallion & Bull (d) Bull & buck

518) First surgical buffalo embryo transfer calf born in Asia at –

(a) NRCC (b) NII
(c) NDRI (d) SAG

519) First non surgical buffalo embryo transfer calf born on –

(a) 4 October 1988 (b) 22nd Dec 1987
(c) 19 March 1988 (d) 16 October 1987

520) The mitochondria are located in spermatozoa–

(a) Apical segment of head (b) Mid–piece
(c) Tail (d) Equatorial segment of head

521) The first embryo transfer was performed in rabbit in the year –

(a) 1650 (b) 1890
(c) 1950 (d) 2000

522) The embryonic origin of ledig cells -

(a) Coelomic cells (b) Primary sex cord
(c) Mesenchymal cells (d) Pronephros

523) The female has two chromosomes, which are

(a) X and X (b) X and Y
(c) X and O (d) XX and Y

524) Antenatal sex can not be determined by performing
(a) Culture of leucocytes
(b) Karyotyping
(c) Fluroscence microscope to detect Y chromosomes
(d) Maternal progestrone level during pregnancy

525) Sperm placed in hypo-tonic solution react by
(a) Swelling (b) Shrinking
(c) No changes (d) All

526) Sperm from follwing organ/ site may not be fertile
(a) Epididymal tail (b) Ampulla
(c) Testicles (d) Epididymal head

527) Karyotyping can be done in cells in foll woing stage of divison
(a) Anaphase (b) Metaphase
(c) P orophase (d) Telophase

528) The F body in the sperm is usally associated with
(a) X- Chromosome (b) Y-Chromosome
(c) Both (d) None

529) X and Y sperm can not be seprated by
(a) Flow sorting by DNA contant
(b) Sephadex column
(c) HY antigen
(d) Dilution with EYC dilutor

530) The following hormone can not be used for ovulation induction therapeutically
(a) Hcg (b) GnRH
(c) Progestrone (d) LH

531) The most common harmone for superovulation is-
(a) PMSG (b) Estrogen
(c) Progestrone (d) PGF2 alpha

532) The life of Corpus l ut eum can be extended by injection of

(a) Inhibin (b) Estradiol 17B
(c) GnRH (d) Progesterone

533) The life of CL is shortered by injection of

(a) Progestron (b) HCG
(c) PGF2 alpha (d) GnRH

534) The Natural leteolytic agent secreted by endometrium

(a) Progestron (b) Estradiol
(c) PGF2 Alpha (d) Relaxin

535) FSH is injected at 12 hrs interval in the morning and evening in divding dose as against EGC, because it has

(a) Shorter half life (b) Longer half life
(c) Antigenic (d) All

536) Super ovulation does not increase normal embryo significantly in

(a) Cow (b) Bitch
(c) Mare (d) Sow

537) Capacitation of sperm occurs in

(a) Testis (b) Epididymis
(c) Ampulla (d) Female reproductive tract

538) Fertilization can not be acertained by following

(a) Penetration of sperm in ooplasm
(b) Pronuclear formation
(c) Blastocyte formation
(d) Presence of cumulus oophrus cell in 4-5 layers

539) Choose a nuclear sperm defect -

(a) Diadem defect (b) Cork-screw sperm
(c) Knobbed defect (d) Dag's defect

540) The Embryo can be transferred to recepient in IVF

(a) Immediately after fertilization
(b) After culturing them in suitable media
(c) After collection of cumulus cells
(d) None

541) Inhibin and Activins are the proteinshormones secreted by

(a) Adrenals (b) Lungs
(c) Heart (d) Gonads

542) Following hormones is /are precursor of Estradiol

(a) Insulin (b) Angiotensin
(c) Androgen (d) Pepsin

543) Estrogen hormone have follwing feedback mechnism

(a) Negative (b) Positive
(c) Both (d) None

544) In Conventional Cryopreservation of embryoes, the embryos are

(a) Equilibrated with freezing media for 20 minutes
(b) Not Equilibriated
(c) Equilibrated for 48 hrs
(d) Equilibrated for 96 hrs

545) In Conventional method of embryo, the other cryoprotectant not used are

(a) Ethylene Glycol (b) DMSO
(c) Aminoacids (d) None

546) In Non Equilibrated Cryopreservation or Vitrification, the embryo

(a) Slowly cooled to -30°C
(b) Directly plugged into LN2 after bried explore at room temprture
(c) Cooled at -96°C
(d) All of them

547) Egg can be denuaded of cumulus cells by enzyme

(a) Amalse (b) Invertase
(c) Hyaluronidase (d) All of them

548) In Intracytoplasmic injection of sperm, the immotile sperm are injected into

(a) Zona Pellucida (b) Perivitelline Space
(c) Dirctly into Vitellus (d) None

549) Synchronization of estrus cannot be not in cattle by alone-

(a) FSH (b) LH

(c) ECG (d) Progestron

550) Transgenic Animals are, in which

(a) Karyotyping has been done

(b) Mitosis has been stopped

(c) Foreign gene has been introduced

(d) No change is done

551) In DNA Microinjection, the gene are

(a) Injected into host genome (b) Gene are activated

(c) Gene are ablated (d) All of them

552) Hatching of blastocytes occurs in cattle

(a) On fertilization (b) 2 days after fertiliztion

(c) 9-11 days after fertilization (d) 15 days after fertilization

553) Cuboni test for pregnancy is performed in

(a) Mare Urine (b) Mare Blood

(c) Mare Serum (b) Mare Milk

554) Cuboni test in mares can be performed for pregnancy diagnosed during

(a) 60-80 days (b) 80-120 days

(c) 150-200 days (d) 200-300 days

555) Pre-estrus bleeding is observed in

(a) Cattle/Buffalo (b) Mare

(c) Sow (d) Bitch

556) Post-estrus bleeding is observed in

(a) Mare (b) Cattle

(c) Bitch (d) Sow

557) Retention of fetal membranes occur in abortion due to

(a) Trichomoniasis (b) Vibrosis

(c) Brucellosis (d) b & c

558) Bilateral Hip flexion posture is also known as
(a) Breech presentation
(b) Nape posture
(c) Dog sitting posture
(d) None

559) The female mammalian reproduction is governed by
(a) Anterior Pituitary
(b) Hypothalamic – pituitary axis
(c) Medulla oblongata
(d) All of the above

560) Post-coital pyometra is commonly observed in –
(a) Brucellosis
(b) Vibriosis
(c) Trichomoniasis
(d) IBR-IPV virus infection

561) The most accurate technique for pregnancy diagnosis in bitches at 20 days of pregnancy-
(a) Cessation of estrus
(b) Abdominal palpatation
(c) Progesterone assay
(d) Ultrasonography

562) Placenta is considered to be retained in bovine if it is not expelled within-
(a) 6-8 hrs
(b) 8-10 hrs
(c) 12-24 hrs
(d) 24-36 hrs

563) Ovulation occurs after end of estrus in -
(a) Bitches
(b) Cows
(c) Goats
(d) Pigs

564) The most common cause of dystocia in sow is –
(a) Primary uterine interia
(b) Secondary uterine interia
(c) Idiopathic uterine interia
(d) Obstetrical disorder

565) A fetal monster characterized by lateral curvature of spine –
(a) Campylorachis scoliosa
(b) Perosomus elumbis
(c) Perosomus horridus
(d) Schistosomus reflex

566) Milk progesterone assay to diagnose pregnancy in cow is done on =
(a) 15 days of post service
(b) 21-24 days of post service
(b) 35 days of post service
(d) 5-10 day of post service

567) Torsion of uterus is most commonly observed in –

(a) Mare (b) Cow
(c) Buffalo (d) Ewe

568) Mid cycle heat in cows is diagnosed by rectal examination by presence of

(a) Well developed follicles (b) Functional C.L.
(c) Regressing C.L (d) Corpus albicans

569) The embryonic origin of Leydig cells

(a) Coelomic cells (b) Primary sex cords
(c) Mesenchymal cells (d) Pronephors

570) The immunoglobulin present in semen is –

(a) Ig G (b) Ig A
(c) IgM (d) None

571) Prostaglandin in male is secreted by –

(a) Prostate (b) Seminal vesicle
(c) Cowper's gland (d) Ampulla

572) The specific staining used for detecting acrosomal sperm defect is –

(a) Eosin –nigrosin staining (b) Giemsa staining
(c) Leishman staining (d) Papnicolou staining

573) Feminizing tumour of testis-

(a) Granulosa cell tumor (b) Sertoli cell tumor
(c) Arrhenoblastoma (d) Leydig cell tumor

574) Non sexual erection of penis is known as –

(a) Pederasty (b) Priaoism
(c) Carnal intercourse (d) Satyiasis

575) A species in which semen is alkaline –

(a) Ram (b) Buck
(c) Boar (d) Bull

576) Enzyme that aids in penetration of spermatozoa by sperm head

(a) Hyaluronidase (b) Acrosin
(c) Lipase (d) Catalase

577) A.I. glass catheter are sterilized by dry heat for half hours at

(a) 100°C (b) 160°C
(c) 200°C (d) 260°C

578) The spermicidal factor in fresh milk –

(a) Phospholipid (b) Lactenin
(c) Lactalbumin (d) Caesin

579) One dose of liquid semen for ideal conception by A. I. in cow should atleast contain motile sperms at a rate of –

(a) 1-15 million (b) 10-15 million
(c) 20-25 million (d) 25-30 million

580) The most commonly recognized disease of the internal genitalia of the bulls-

(a) Prostatitis (b) Vesiculitis
(c) Ampullities (d) Epididymitis

581) The repeat breeder cow has an estrus cycle length of –

(a) Long duration (b) Short duration
(c) Normal length (d) Split heat

582) An inter estrus length of 30 -35 days is an indication of –

(a) Delayed ovulation (b) 3rd degree endometritis
(c) Early embryonic death (d) Failure of fertilization

583) Aplasia of one horn of uterus is termed as –

(a) Uterine hypoplasia (b) Uterine unicornis
(c) Uterine didelphis (d) Uterine agenesis

584) The spilling of the contents of cortical granules into peri vitelline space is responsible for

(a) Acrosomal reaction (b) Polyspermy
(c) Zona reaction (d) Parthenogenesis

585) Capacitation is accomplished by binding of sperm with
- (a) Glyceryl phosphoryl choline
- (b) Glycosaminoglycans
- (c) Phospho lipids
- (d) Lecithin

586) The inflammation of the outer most layer of uterus is called as-
- (a) Endometritis
- (b) Perimetritis
- (c) Parametritis
- (d) Metritis

587) Sexually deformed female partner of a hetero sexual twin in cattle is called as-
- (a) Mosaic
- (b) Hermaphrodite
- (c) Bull dog
- (d) Freemartin

588) Harrops model of artificial vagina is associated with semen collection from-
- (a) Stallion
- (b) Boar
- (c) Cock
- (d) Dog

589) Robertsonian translocation in bovines involves the chromosomes
- (a) 1 & 29
- (b) 2 & 21
- (c) 7 & 32
- (d) 5 & 15

590) The uterine infection accompanied by accumulation of pus in uterus and anesturm-
- (a) 1st degree endometritis
- (b) 2nd degree endometritis
- (c) 3rd degree endometritis
- (d) Hydroma

591) Casting of calf bed is –
- (a) Uterine torsion
- (b) Postpartum uterine eversion
- (c) Prepartum cervico-vaginal prolapsed
- (d) Uterine rupture

592) Metestral bleeding seen in cattle is due to –
- (a) Estrogen stimulation
- (b) Estrogen withdrawal
- (c) Progesterone withdrawal
- (d) Progesterone stimulation

593) A test to assay patency of salpinx in bovines

(a) Cuboni test (b) P. S. P. test
(c) White side test (d) Aschiem Zonak test

594) A condition where semen sample contains reduced number of sperms

(a) Azoospermia (b) Athenozoospermia
(c) Oligozoospermia (d) Necrospermia

595) Most effective drug to treat bovine fetal mummification –

(a) Dexamethasone (b) Progesterone
(c) Prostaglandin (d) Oxytocin

596) A diluents in which Nitrogen is bubbled to maintain pH –

(a) C M E (b) Caprogen
(c) IVT (d) Caw

597) Durg of choice in primary uterine interia –

(a) Estrogen (b) Progestrone
(c) Oxytocin (d) hCG

598) Intra uterine death of fetus followed by absorption of fetal fluids may lead to –

(a) Fetal Maceration (b) Fetal Mummification
(c) Hydramnion (d) Hydro allantois

599) The cavernous structure that closes the neck of the urinary bladder during sexual excitement which prevents urination during ejaculation-

(a) Corpus cavernosum penis (b) Corpus spongiosum penis
(c) Colliculus seminalis (d) Corpus fibrinosum penis

600) The first water bag expelled during parturition

(a) Allanto chorion (b) Allantois
(c) Amnion (d) Chorion

601) The causative agent for epizootic bovine abortion –

(a) Chlamydia (b) Brucella
(c) Mycoplasma (d) IBR-IPV

602) Rosette Inhibition test for pregnancy diagnosis is for detection of –
(a) hCG (b) EPF
(c) b-PAG (d) alpha interferon

603) Total head abnormalities of bull semen sample should not exceed-
(a) 10% (b) 5%
(c) 15% (d) 20%

604) The technique used for collection of oocytes from live animals (Full)
(a) TVOR (b) MOET
(c) IVP (d) Slicing

605) This is an anti-prolactin agents -
(a) Progynon (b) Proluton
(c) Bromocryptin (d) Lutalyse

606) Postural abnormalities of head and neck of fetus are most commonly observed in dystocia of –
(a) Cow (b) Mare
(c) Sheep (d) Goat

607) A patent product containing natural PGF2 alpha –
(a) Estrumate (b) Clofert
(c) Lutalyse (d) Iliren

608) Which is the precursor for spermatozoa acrosome-
(a) Chromatoid body (b) Golgi apparatus
(c) Mitochondria (d) Ribosome

609) In addition to spermatozoa which of the following may be seen in stained semen smears
(a) Spermatids (b) Medusa cells
(c) Squamousa epithelial cells (d) All of them

610) The intra tubular germ mother cells are -
(a) Spermatogonia (b) Sertoli cells
(c) Leydig cells (d) Spermatids

611) Estrogen is secreted by which of the following

(a) Zona pellucid
(b) Membrane granulose
(c) Theca interna
(d) Theca externa

612) Swiss cheese appearance of endometrium is seen in –

(a) Luteal cyst
(b) Follicular cyst
(c) Both a & b
(d) Par-ovarian cyst

613) Cloudburst is associated with pseudo pregnancy –

(a) Goat
(b) Horse
(c) Pig
(d) Dog

614) Speices in which luteolysis is transported locally, but not exclusive to the adjacent ovary -

(a) Equine
(b) Caprine
(c) Swine
(d) Bovine

615) Surgical correction employed for chronic prolapsed of vagina and wind sucking -

(a) Episiotomy
(b) Caslicks operation
(c) Zepps
(d) Canthotomy

616) "Casting of calf bed" is a colloquial term given for –

(a) Prolapse of bladder
(b) Prolapse of uterus
(c) R. O. P.
(d) Lochial discharge

617) Precurser of prostaglandins –

(a) Cholestrol
(b) Arachidonic Acid
(c) Benzoic acid
(d) Caproic acid

618) Hormone secrete from pars intermedia

(a) TSH
(b) MSH
(c) CRH
(d) ACTH

619) The pigment 'uteroverdin' is associated with placenta of –

(a) Swine
(b) Equine
(c) Canine
(d) Bovine

620) Number of follicular waves commonly seen in estrus cycle of cow-

(a) 1-2
(b) 2-3
(c) 3-5
(d) 4-5

621) Which is a mono-estrus animal -

(a) Cat
(b) Horse
(c) Bitch
(d) Camel

622) Phantom (Pseudo) pregnancy in bitches is due to action of which hormone -

(a) Estrogen
(b) Progesterone
(c) Prolactin
(d) Oxytocin

623) Non hormonal method of synchronization in ewes-

(a) Prolactin
(b) Weaning
(c) Artificial light
(d) Pheromones

624) Survivability of spermatozoa in reproductive tract of bitches –

(a) 24 hrs
(b) 8 hrs
(c) 2-3 days
(d) 4-7 days

625) Site of A. I. with frozen semen in pigs –

(a) Intracervical
(b) Intrauterine
(c) Anterior vagina
(d) All of them

626) The best way of packing the sperm for freezing is in -

(a) Glass ampoules
(b) Pellets
(c) Straws
(d) Plastic capsules

627) The key factor that determines shedding of after birth is –

(a) First stage labor
(b) Placental maturity
(c) Abdominal contraction
(d) Second stage labor

628) Shortening the estrus cycle is one of the approaches to treat endometritis, how does it help ?

(a) Enhance uterine defense
(b) Cleanses the uterus
(c) Flushes the uterus
(d) Absorbs contant

629) A non invasive technique to prevent recurring geneital prolapses is–
(a) Hind limb on elevated plateform
(b) Rope truse
(c) Medicinal therapy
(d) Buhner's technique

630) Which one of the statement in respect of the application of progesterone in clinical practice is true-
(a) It prevents prolpase
(b) Its application has no rationality
(c) It stops threatened abortions with no complications
(d) It controls genital prolapse

631) Per vaginal delivery of oversized fetus is effected by –
(a) Slow and gradual but simultaneous traction on both limbs
(b) Disengage limbs and traction on other
(c) Place the dam on its dorsum
(d) Alternative traction on limbs

632) A pathognomic symptom of nymphomania –
(a) Arching of the spine
(b) Pseudo hump
(c) Bowed legs
(d) Sterility hump

633) The circulating concentration of that hormone increase upon clitorial stimulation (massage)
(a) Histamine
(b) Oxytocin
(c) PGF2 alpha
(d) Estradiol

634) Site of A.I. with frozen semen in pigs-
(a) Intracervical
(b) Intrauterine
(c) Anterior Vagina
(d) All of the above

635) Accessory gland present in cats, but not in dogs -
(a) Bubourethal
(b) Prostate
(c) Seminal Vesicle
(d) None of the above

636) Spermatogenesis is regulated by which of the hormones-
(a) FSH
(b) LH
(c) Testosterone
(d) Estrogen

637) Collaginase, used for the treatment of retention of foetal membrane is administrated through-

(a) Intramusular route
(b) Intravenous route
(c) Intra uterine
(d) Retained umbilical cord

638) Which of the following is congenital sperm detected affecting the acrosome-

(a) Dag defect
(b) Decapitate defect
(c) Pseudo droplet
(d) Knobbed sperm defect

639) Temperature of liquid nitrogen is -

(a) -180°C
(b) -196°C
(c) -79°C
(d) -179°C

640) In cattle, embryo moves from the oviduct to uterus –

(a) 2-3 days of ovulation
(b) 3-4 days of ovulation
(c) 5-6 days of ovulation
(d) 7-8 days of ovulation

641) The earliest day by which pregnancy can be distinguished in cattle by B-mode real time ultrasonography-

(a) 3 days
(b) 6 days
(c) 9 days
(d) 19 days

642) Stain used for flow cytometric sorting of spermatozoa –

(a) Eosin-Nigrosin
(b) Giemsa stain
(c) FITC
(d) Hoechs 33342

643) Hermaphodism is more common in-

(a) Caprine
(b) Dog
(c) Horse
(d) Cattle

644) An anomaly in cattle in which the fetus lacks coccygeal vertebrae and has deformed sacral vertebrae with a sunken perineal region -

(a) Spinabifida
(b) Hemivertebrea
(c) Schistosomus reflexus
(d) Perosomus acaudatus

645) True extauterine pregnancy is seen in –

(a) Human
(b) Dogs
(c) Swine
(d) Cattle

646) Maternal recognition of pregnancy starts in cattle by –
(a) 16-17 days (b) 12-13 days
(c) 20-22 days (d) 6-7 days

647) Cervical star is associated with pregnancy in-
(a) Cows (b) Sow
(c) Heifer (d) Mare

648) The Ideal duration of dry period in a pregnant cow-
(a) 30 days (b) 45 days
(c) 60 days (d) 90 days

649) Hook head spermatozoa are characteristic of –
(a) Cock (b) Rat
(c) Guinea pig (d) Duck

650) The substrate for endogenous respiration of spermatozoa –
(a) Glucose (b) Fructose
(c) Plasmalogen (d) Sucrose

651) White side test for the diagnosis of endometritis is done by using-
(a) 10% Egg white (b) 5% NAOH
(c) 10% Nacl (d) 5% NaHCo3

652) Du Vigeneaud got the Nobel Prize in 1955 for his research on –
(a) Oxytocin (b) Progesterone
(c) Estrogen (d) Prostaglandin

653) The precursor for the hormone melatonin is the amino acid –
(a) Tryptophan (b) Tyrosin
(c) Arginine (d) Lysin

654) The release of formed germ cells into the lumen of seminiferous tubule is known as –
(a) Spermatocytocytogenesis (b) Spematogenesis
(c) Spermiogenesis (d) Spermiation

655) The transport time for bull spermatozoa through epididymis-

(a) 3 days (b) 11 days
(c) 17 days (d) 21 days

656) Presence of cytoplasmic droplet in a significance number of spermatozoa is a sign of immaturity except in-

(a) Boar (b) Dog
(c) Bull (d) Buck

657) Which of the following statement is flase with respect to cryptorchidism

(a) The thermal need of testis are not maintained
(b) Normal spermatogenic function is not possible
(c) Endocrine function of testis is impaired
(d) More or less normal sexual desire is exhibited

658) The major portion of extra gonadal sperm reserves of ruminants is found in -

(a) Caput epididymis (b) Corpus epididymis
(c) Cauda epididymis (d) Ampulla

659) The only accessory gland present in a male dog is -

(a) Seminal vesicle (b) Prostate
(c) Bulbourethral gland (d) Ampulla

660) Flutamide is-

(a) Antiandrogen (b) Antiestrogen
(c) Antiprolactin (d) Antiprogesterone

661) Drug of choice for bovine pyometra-

(a) Progesterone (b) Ethinyl estradiol
(c) Prostaglandin (d) Cabergoline

662) Foot nape posture is most common in -

(a) Eqiune (b) Bovine
(c) Caprine (d) Porcine

663) A cryprotectant used in frozen semen production
(a) TRIS (b) Fructose
(c) Citric acid (d) Glycerol

664) The pelvic inlet is more round in -
(a) Cow (b) Ewe
(c) Mare (d) Sow

665) Immobilization reflex and lordosis are characteristics sign of estrus–
(a) Mare (b) Cat
(c) Rabbit (d) Sow

666) Block to polyspermy is achieved by –
(a) Acrosomal reaction
(b) Cortical reaction
(c) Enzymes produced by spermatozoa
(d) All of them

667) The function of sertoli cells are –
(a) Production of androgen binding protein and FSH
(b) Production of estrogen and androgen
(c) Production of estrogen and androgen binding protein
(d) Conversion of testosterone to dihydro-testosterone

668) Inhibin exerts negative feed back over hypothalamusand-pituitary-axis to control the release of –
(a) FSH & LH (b) LH alone
(c) FSH alone (d) FSH & Prolactin

669) Placenta is considered to be retained in cattle if it is not expelled within-
(a) 12 hrs (b) 24 hrs
(c) 48 hrs (d) 72 hrs

670) The ovaries affected with total hypoplasia will appear –
(a) Pea shaped
(b) Bean shaped
(c) Flat, shrunken and shriveled with longitudinal furrows
(d) Heart shaped

671) The ideal treatment for follicular cyst and nymphomania is -
(a) Manual rupture
(b) LH or LHRH
(c) LH or LHRH followed by prostaglandin on 10th day
(d) FSH & Prolactin

672) The normal duration of second stage of parturition in mare is -
(a) 20 minutes (b) 2 hrs
(c) 4 hrs (d) 8 hrs

673) Pregnanacy can be correctly diagnosed in goats at 2 months by
(a) Abdominal palpation (b) Radiology
(c) Bimanual palpation method (d) ELISA

674) The attainment of puberty in cattle is more correlated with-
(a) Age (b) Body weight
(c) Enzymatic changes in blood (d) None

675) Clitoris will develope from -
(a) Mullerian duct (b) Urogeneital tract
(c) Genital tubercle (d) Urethral fold

676) The peptide secreted by the ovary is -
(a) Estrogen (b) Progesterone
(c) Oxytocin (d) F. S. H.

677) Post coital pyometra is commonly observed in -
(a) Brucellosis (b) Vibriosis
(c) Trichomoniasis (d) IBR- IPV

678) Persistent penile frenulum will result in-
(a) Ventral deviation of penis (b) Lateral deviation of penis
(c) Spiral deviation of penis (d) All of them

679) Spermiogenesis is regulated by which of the hormones-
(a) FSH (b) LH
(c) Testosterone (d) Estrogen

680) Maturation and fertilization ability of spermatozoa are occurring at–

(a) Rete testis (b) Epididymis
(c) Seminiferous tubules (d) Ampulla

681) Pregnancy diagnosis is much more accurate per rectum during which trimester of gestation in cattle –

(a) First trimester (b) Second trimester
(c) Third trimester (d) Any trimester

682) In which species of animal the season and photoperiod, both affects the onset of puberty –

(a) Sheep (b) Pig
(c) Cattle (d) Buffalo

683) Sexual differentiation in bovines occur by –

(a) 60 days (b) 45 days
(c) 30 days (d) 15 days

684) It is the precursor for spermatozoa acrosome –

(a) Chomatil body (b) Golgi body
(c) Ribosome (d) Mitochondria

685) It is a reversible testicular condition

(a) Hypoplasia (b) Degeneration
(c) Fibrosis (d) Cryptorchidism

686) The species that produced semen with large volume and low sperm concentration –

(a) Bovine (b) Caprine
(c) Stallion (d) Canine

687) The first sign of testicular degeneration is the presence of -

(a) Loose heads (b) Tail defects
(c) Dead cells (d) Immotile cells

688) The initial evaluation of semen is carried out at –

(a) 40°C (b) 25°C
(c) 30-35°C (d) 42°C

689) The method commonly used for studying the sperm tail abnormalities is –

(a) H & E (b) Eosin & Nigrosine
(c) Formal saline (d) Williams

690) The animal that has calved twice or more is called as –

(a) Uniparous (b) Multiparous
(c) Pluriparous (d) Primiparous

691) The percent of eosin present in vita stain is –

(a) 1.67 (b) 1.0
(c) 0.67 (d) 16.7

692) The arrangement that prevents the entry of certain substance and allows the free passage of others is known as –

(a) Tunica albuginea (b) Myloid layer
(c) Blood – testis barrier (d) Soermatids

693) The form of infertility caused by affections of locomotor system is –

(a) Lack of sex drive (b) Impotentia cocundi
(c) Impotenia gnenrandi (d) Transient

694) The fertility of a bilaterally cryptorchid animals is –

(a) Reduced (b) Optimum
(c) Maintained (d) Zero

695) Which is the precursor of spermatozoa acrosome -

(a) Chromatid body (b) Golgi apparatus
(c) Mitocondria (d) Ribosome

696) The main hormone responsible for relaxation of pelvic ligaments is–

(a) Relaxin (b) Prostaglandins
(c) Progesterone (d) Estrogen

697) Morula has _____ number of cells

(a) 16-32 (b) 4-8
(c) 2-4 (d) 64-128

698) Biological half life of LH is –

(a) 30 min (b) 70 min
(c) 15 min (d) 45 min

699) Rigs are commonly a condition observed in –

(a) Stallion (b) Bull
(c) Dog (d) Boar

700) The primary abnormality of spermatozoa is –

(a) Pyriform head (b) Loss head
(c) Coiled mid piece (d) None

ANSWER KEYS

1. (b) 15-17 days of gestation
2. (c) Corpus luteum verum
3. (a) Ovarian Steriod Hormone
4. (c) Placenta
5. (b) Leydig cells
6. (a) Poor egg quality
7. (c) Trichomoniasis
8. (c) Super ovulation
9. (c) 30-48 hrs
10. (a) 8-10 hrs
11. (b) 13
12. (b) 25-30
13. (b) 148 days
14. (a) Trophoblastic cells
15. (d) Diestrus
16. (c) Fornix
17. (b) Synthetic androgen
18. (d) Prolactin
19. (a) Bitches
20. (a) Fertagyl
21. (a) Anovulation
22. (c) PGF_2 alpha
23. (a) Estrus detection
24. (d) 4-7 days
25. (c) Rabbit
26. (a) Swine
27. (c) 150-200 days

28. (c) Mare
29. (a) Nutritional deficiency
30. (c) Local hormone
31. (a) Mare
32. (d) Sow
33. (a) Mare
34. (d) 12-14 hrs after the end of oestrus
35. (c) Progesterone
36. (d) Sheep
37. (c) 40-120 days
38. (d) FSH
39. (d) More than 100000
40. (a) Bitch
41. (b) Cow
42. (b) Mare
43. (a) 6-8 hours
44. (b) 16-24 hours
45. (d) All of the above
46. (c) Kangaroo
47. (c) Opossum
48. (c) Dog
49. (c) Mare
50. (b) Protein hormone
51. (c) Induction of parturition
52. (c) Super ovulation
53. (c) Trichomoniasis
54. (b) Brucellosis
55. (b) Mare
56. (c) Mare

57. (b) Progesterone
58. (b) Human placenta
59. (c) Dead fetus
60. (b) Corpus luteum
61. (c) Theca interna cells
62. (a) Facilitate removal of micro-organism
63. (a) Ovarian steroid hormones
64. (d) Equine placenta
65. (c) Cerebral cortex
66. (b) Mare
67. (d) 300-310 days
68. (c) 330-340 days
69. (b) 56-65 days
70. (d) 333-430 days
71. (d) 113-115 days
72. (d) 208 -240 days
73. (c) 140-155 days
74. (c) 105-112 days
75. (c) 615 -650 days
76. (b) 8-16 days
77. (c) Camel
78. (c) 9-15 days
79. (c) 35 months
80. (b) 12-18 months
81. (b) 10-24 months
82. (a) 5-8 months
83. (b) 1-2days before end of oestrus
84. (c) 36-48 h. after the onset of estrum
85. (b) 4-13day

86. (a) 1-2 day after the onset of estrum
87. (b) 40 months
88. (b) 18 months
89. (c) 45 months
90. (b) 30 months
91. (b) Mare
92. (a) Interferon tau
93. (a) Bitch
94. (b) During 2nd month of pregnancy
95. (a) 2-3 days after its formation
96. (b) 40-120 days after service
97. (c) Boar
98. (b) 12-13 days
99. (b) 12 days
100. (c) 14-16 days
101. (d) 40-45 days
102. (c) Day 18
103. (b) 15-16 days
104. (c) 25-38 days
105. (c) Granulosa cells
106. (b) Sialic acid
107. (c) 6-8 days after ovulation
108. (d) Inter-estrus period
109. (a) Prigma
110. (a) Brucella
111. (b) Inhibin
112. (b) Adrenal cortex
113. (b) Chlomiphene
114. (b) Glycoprotein

115. (a) Sheep, goat and horse
116. (a) FSH
117. (c) Prostaglandin
118. (d) Progesterone
119. (c) Placenta
120. (c) Estrogen
121. (b) Progesterone
122. (b) Regression of corpus luteum
123. (b) Utero-ovarian pathway
124. (a) Bitch
125. (a) Cow
126. (d) 80-120
127. (c) Cow
128. (d) Diestrus
129. (a) Bitch
130. (c) Both a and b
131. (d) All of the above
132. (c) Progesterone
133. (c) ACTH
134. (b) Intra venous
135. (c) Urine of pregnant mare
136. (c) Bitch
137. (b) Coitus
138. (a) Post coital pyometra
139. (b) Luteal phase
140. (a) Multiple ovulation and embryo transfer
141. (a) Hormonal derangement of LH
142. (a) Early pregnancy diagnosis
143. (c) 17- ketosteroids

144. (c) Uterus
145. (a) Mare
146. (c) Abnormal presentation, position and posture
147. (a) Diffuse
148. (a) 5 to 15 days after foaling
149. (c) Canine
150. (d) Prolactin
151. (a) Anovulation
152. (d) Less than one hour
153. (c) Rabbit
154. (a) Swine
155. (b) 8-16 days of gestation
156. (d) 5-7 months of gestations
157. (b) Breech presentation
158. (b) Hormonal Imbalance
159. (b) Progesterone
160. (c) Ring womb
161. (d) 7.2-7.6
162. (b) 270-310 m OSM/kg
163. (c) Embryo collection
164. (c) 6-8 ml
165. (c) Progesterone
166. (d) During 3rd trimester
167. (a) Dead fetus
168. (a) Anterior longitudinal
169. (c) Brucellosis
170. (a) Cow
171. (a) Mare
172. (a) Hydrocephalus

173. (b) Doe
174. (c) Casting of calfbed
175. (c) Buffalo
176. (b) Placentome
177. (c) Post partum paralysis
178. (d) Whelping
179. (d) Cervix and prepubic tendon
180. (c) Prolapse of uterus
181. (d) 40 days
182. (c) Retention of fetal membranes
183. (c) Ring womb
184. (c) PCL
185. (b) Mare
186. (b) Brucellosis
187. (c) Canine
188. (c) Buffalo
189. (c) Uterine inertia
190. (b) Progesterone
191. (a) 5-12 days post partum
192. (b) Fetal cortisol
193. (b) Mare
194. (a) Hormonal dysfunction
195. (c) Hydrometra
196. (b) Cotyledonary
197. (d) Man
198. (c) Dog
199. (a) Buffaloes
200. (d) Discoid
201. (a) Man

202. (a) 1-4 hours
203. (b) During 2nd month of pregnancy
204. (a) 2-3 days after its formation
205. (d) 40-45 days
206. (c) Day 18
207. (b) 15-16 days
208. (c) 25-38 days
209. (a) Increased fetal production of corticoids
210. (d) Estrogen, relaxin, cortisol and prostaglandin
211. (d) Bitch
212. (a) 17 alpha Hydroxylase
213. (d) Progesterone
214. (c) Placenta
215. (c) Estrogen
216. (d) 80-120
217. (c) Cow
218. (d) Diestrus
219. (b) Mare
220. (c) Both a and b
221. (d) All of the above
222. (a) Estrogen
223. (a) Estrogen
224. (d) All of the above
225. (a) 30-40 days of gestation
226. (c) Forward and downward in the abdominal cavity
227. (a) Mare
228. (d) 100 days and above
229. (a) Serum of pregnant mare
230. (d) All of the above

231. (d) All of the above
232. (d) Panting
233. (b) During second stage of parturition
234. (b) Stillbirth
235. (a) Abortion
236. (a) Hematinic
237. (a) Fetal mummification
238. (b) Peptide
239. (b) Papyraceous type
240. (a) Same direction
241. (a) Rolling of the dam
242. (a) Abnormal presentation, position and posture
243. (a) Cow
244. (d) Both b and c
245. (d) both a & b
246. (c) Discoidal
247. (c) Endoderm
248. (a) Endoderm and splanchnopleuric mesoderm
249. (d) Both a and b
250. (a) Cattle
251. (a) Hydrocephalus
252. (d) Syndactilism
253. (a) Schistosomus reflesus
254. (a) Traction
255. (c) Repellor
256. (a) Repulsion
257. (a) Mutation
258. (c) Repulsion
259. (a) Rotation

260. (d) All of the
261. (b) Progesterone
262. (d) Oxytocin
263. (d) Fallopian tube
264. (d) Camel
265. (d) Camel
266. (b) 310 days
267. (a) 62 days
268. (b) Priapism
269. (a) Genital prolapse
270. (d) After end of estrus
271. (c) Late estrus
272. (c) Late estrus
273. (a) Early estrus
274. (c) 24-30 hours after coitus
275. (a) 26
276. (b) Leydig cells
277. (c) Stallion
278. (c) 200-300 million/ml
279. (d) Oviduct
280. (a) Cattle
281. (a) 500 million/ml
282. (b) Testicular Degeneration
283. (b) Epididymes
284. (b) Baltelk
285. (a) 16″ x 2.5″
286. (b) Epididymes
287. (d) Mishandling of semen
288. (a) Erick Bloom

289. (b) Diadem defect
290. (b) Caput epididymes
291. (a) 3-5 minutes
292. (b) Teratozoo spermia
293. (a) Norman *et al.*
294. (b) EYC
295. (d) 1152 mm
296. (d) 2-5% of the semen by volume
297. (d) Dog
298. (c) Anterior cervix
299. (c) Spermatic artery
300. (b) Dog
301. (c) Cat
302. (a)Ram
303. (b) 7%
304. (a) 3.5 -4monthsmonthsof gestation
305. (d) 9-11 months of gestation
306. (b) 70 days of gestation
307. (d) 5 days after birth
308. (d) 5000 meters
309. (c) 150 meters
310. (b) Sertoli cells
311. (c) 30 meters
312. (a) 20 meters
313. (b) 50 meters
314. (a) 10 days
315. (c) 9-12 days
316. (b) Stallion
317. (c) Boar

318. (b) Bull
319. (d) Boar
320. (b) Dog
321. (b) Ram
322. (b) Sheep and goat
323. (a) Stallion
324. (b) Lazzaro Spallanzani
325. (c) Sampat Kumaran
326. (a) Case
327. (c) Baltelli
328. (c) Komorou
329. (d) 85-98%
330. (c) 10%
331. (a) 2-5%
332. (b) 31-38%
333. (c) 31-36%
334. (d) 31-32%
335. (b) Fructose
336. (d) 500 mg/100 ml
337. (c) 30-48 hours
338. (a) Immunosuppressive effect
339. (d) 72-120 hours
340. (c) 30-48 hours
341. (c) 24-72 hours
342. (d) Swine
343. (c) 36-48 h. after the onset of estrum
344. (a) 1-2 d. after the onset of estrum
345. (c) 1000 million per ml
346. (c) 900 million per ml

347. (b) 400 million per ml
348. (d) 2000 million per ml
349. (b) 300 million per ml
350. (a) 300 million per ml
351. (a) 150 million per ml
352. (b) 12-18 months
353. (c) 24-30 months
354. (b) 18-24 months
355. (a) 7-8 months
356. (a) 6-7 months
357. (a) 8-10 months
358. (b) 5 degree centigrade
359. (d) Indefinite
360. (c) 285 milliosmols
361. (c) Neutral pH
362. (d) All of the above
363. (d) Salt and sugar solution
364. (b) Cervix
365. (b) 1951
366. (a) Polge
367. (b) Danish
368. (c) -15 to -60°C
369. (c) Both a and b
370. (a) Lctenin
371. (b) 92-95 degree Celsius for 10 minutes
372. (b) Have better buffering capacity
373. (a) Increased semen volume
374. (b) 4hours at 5 degree Celsius
375. (d) All of the above

376. (d) All of the above
377. (c) Large epididymal sperm reserve
378. (a) Intra uterine
379. (d) Equine
380. (d) Sulfonamide
381. (c) Sunlight
382. (a) Swab method
383. (a) Adverse effect on the quality of semen
384. (b) AV Lewenhock
385. (b) Creating intracellular equilibration
386. (a) Riboflavin
387. (a) Primary abnormalities
388. (c) 30-40 cm
389. (d) 50-55 cm
390. (b) 20-25 cm
391. (c) Both a and b
392. (a) 1:4
393. (c) 5-16 days of cycle
394. (d) Bulbo-urethral gland
395. (d) Boar
396. (c) Boar
397. (c) AV Method
398. (a) EYC dilutor
399. (a) 20
400. (c) Uterus
401. (a) 1ml
402. (d) 250 million / dose
403. (a) Cu & Fe
404. (d) Both a & b

405. (c) Epididymis
406. (a) 70 percent
407. (c) Palace dairy farm Mysore
408. (b) Neck
409. (c) 9+9+2
410. (d) 11+2
411. (a) 66 micron in bull, 68 micron in ram and boar
412. (a) Proximal centriole
413. (b) Alkaline
414. (b) 15-18°C
415. (a) Ergothionine
416. (b) Bull
417. (d) Ergothionine
418. (a) Glucose
419. (d) Seminal Vasiculitis
420. (c) 42-45°C
421. (c) G. Amenta
422. (b) Seminal vesicle
423. (b) Tunica vesculosa
424. (d) Peritoneal fold that holds the fetal epididymis in place
425. (a) Wolffian duct
426. (a) FSH
427. (a) Parkes
428. (a) Polge
429. (c) 1949
430. (b) Mare
431. (a) Flushing
432. (d) Equitoria
433. (d) Dynein

434. (c) Inositol
435. (a) Early Embryonic Mortality
436. (b) 7 percent
437. (b) Stallion
438. (c) Bull
439. (b) High flanker
440. (d) 80-90 percent
441. (a) Estrogen
442. (c) Pear shaped
443. (d) Dog
444. (b) Paraphimosis
445. (a) Bull
446. (c) Rainbow deviation
447. (d) Dog
448. (c) Scrotum
449. (b) Osmotic pressure regulator
450. (b) 10
451. (a) Boar
452. (d) Boar
453. (a) Bull
454. (a) Stallion
455. (b) Bull
456. (d) Stallion
457. (b) Boar
458. (a) 70 percent
459. (b) 50 percent
460. (b) 70 percent
461. (a) 55 percent
462. (b) 20 million motile sperms

463. (c) Poultry
464. (d) Man
465. (b) 100-250 million
466. (b) Middle estrous
467. (c) Late estrous
468. (a) 70-120 hours
469. (a) Early estrous
470. (b) Middle estrous
471. (a) Early estrous
472. (b) Middle estrous
473. (c) Leeuwenhock
474. (b) 1890
475. (c) Walter Heape
476. (a) Mare
477. (d) Sow
478. (a) Mare
479. (d) Hysterectomy
480. (c) Hereditary disease of the embryo
481. (d) Killing ova
482. (c) Back cross
483. (c) Cryptorchidism
484. (c) 17- ketosteroids
485. (a) Sertoli cell tumor
486. (c) Very few days
487. (d) Oxytocin
488. (c) Mare
489. (c) UK
490. (c) NII
491. (d) SAG

492. (b) 22nd Dec 1987
493. (a) Sheep, goat and horse
494. (d) Indefinite
495. (c) 285 milliosmols
496. (c) Neutral pH
497. (d) All of the above
498. (d) Bilateral testicular aplasia
499. (a) Dogs
500. (d) Cervix and prepubic tendon
501. (c) Ruminants
502. (a) Chorionic girdle (fetal origin)
503. (c) Areolae
504. (a) Period of embryo
505. (b) Leptospirosis
506. (d) Retained umbilical cord
507. (a) Stallion
508. (d) Stallion
509. (b) Sow
510. (a) Slightly acidic
511. (d) 1996
512. (c) Hans sperman
513. (b) Madan *et al.*
514. (b) Kumaran
515. (a) Trichomoniasis
516. (b) (b) Brucellosis
517. (b) Buck & Stallion
518. (d) SAG
519. (b) 22nd Dec 1987
520. (b) Mid -piece

521. (b) 1890
522. (c) Mesenchymal cells
523. (a) X and X
524. (d) Maternal progestrone level during pregnancy
525. (a) Swelling
526. (c) Testicles
527. (b) Metaphase
528. (b) Y- Chromosome
529. (d) Dilution with EYC dilutor
530. (c) Progestrone
531. (a) PMSG
532. (d) Progestron
533. (c) PGF2 alpha
534. (c) PGF2 Alpha
535. (a) Shorter half life
536. (d) Sow
537. (d) Female reproductive tract
538. (d) Presence of cumulus oophrus cell in 4-5 layers
539. (a) Diadem defect
540. (b) After culturing them in suitable media
541. (d) Gonads
542. (c) Androgen
543. (c) Both
544. (a) Equilibrated with freezing media for 20 minutes
545. (b) DMSO
546. (b) Directly piuged into LN2 after bried explore at room temprture
547. (c). Hyaluronidase
548. (c) Dirctly into Vitellus
549. (b) LH

550. (c) Foreign gene has been introduced
551. (a) Gene are injected into host genome
552. (c) 9-11 days after fertilization
553. (a) Mare Urine
554. (c) 150-200 days
555. (d) Bitch
556. (b) Cattle/Buffalo
557. (c) Brucellosis
558. (a) Breech presentation
559. (b) Hypothalamic – pituitary axis
560. (c) Trichomoniasis
561. (d) Ultrasonography
562. (c) 12-24 hrs
563. (b) Cows
564. (b) Secondary uterine interia
565. (a) Campylorachis scoliosa
566. (b) 21-24 days of post service
567. (c) Buffalo
568. (b) Functional C.L.
569. (c) Mesenchymal cells
570. (b) Ig A
571. (b) Seminal vesicle
572. (b) Giemsa staining
573. (b) Sertoli cell tumor
574. (b) Priaoism
575. (c) Boar
576. (b) Acrosin
577. (b) 160°C
578. (b) Lactenin

579. (b) 10 -15 million
580. (b) Vesiculitis
581. (c) Normal length
582. (c) Early embryonic death
583. (b) Uterine unicornis
584. (c) Zona reaction
585. (b) Glycosaminoglycans
586. (b) Perimetritis
587. (d) Freemartin
588. (d) Dog
589. (a) 1 & 29
590. (c) 3rd degree endometritis
591. (b) Postpartum uterine eversion
592. (b) Estrogen withdrawal
593. (b) P. S. P. test
594. (c) Oligozoospermia
595. (c) Prostaglandin
596. (b) Caprogen
597. (c) Oxytocin
598. (b) Fetal Mummification
599. (c) Colliculus seminalis
600. (a) Allanto chorion
601. (a) Chlamydia
602. (b) EPF
603. (b) 5%
604. (a) TVOR
605. (c) Bromocryptin
606. (b) Mare
607. (c) Lutalyse

608. (b) Golgi apparatus
609. (d) All of them
610. (b) Sertoli cells
611. (c) Theca interna
612. (b) Follicular cyst
613. (a) Goat
614. (c) Swine
615. (b) Caslicks operation
616. (b) Prolapse of uterus
617. (b) Arachidonic Acid
618. (b) MSH
619. (c) Canine
620. (b) 2-3
621. (c) Bitch
622. (c) Prolactin
623. (c) Artificial light
624. (d) 4-7 days
625. (b) Intrauterine
626. (c) Straws
627. (b) Placental maturity
628. (a) Enhance uterine defense
629. (a) Hind limb on elevated plateform
630. (b) It's application has no ralionality
631. (d) Alternative traction on limbs
632. (d) Sterility hump
633. (b) Oxytocin
634. (b) Intrauterine
635. (a) Bubourethal
636. (a) FSH